Algorithms for Obstetrics and Gynaecology

Algorithms for Obstetrics and Gynaecology

Edited by

Sambit Mukhopadhyay

Consultant Obstetrician and Gynaecologist,
Norfolk and Norwich University Hospital,
Norwich, UK

Edward Morris

Consultant Obstetrician and Gynaecologist,
Norfolk and Norwich University Hospital,
Norwich, UK

Sabaratnam Arulkumaran

Professor Emeritus of Obstetrics and Gynaecology,
St George's University of London,
London, UK

OXFORD
UNIVERSITY PRESS

OXFORD
UNIVERSITY PRESS

Great Clarendon Street, Oxford, OX2 6DP,
United Kingdom

Oxford University Press is a department of the University of Oxford.
It furthers the University's objective of excellence in research, scholarship,
and education by publishing worldwide. Oxford is a registered trade mark of
Oxford University Press in the UK and in certain other countries

First Edition published in 2014

Impression: 1

Published in the United States of America by Oxford University Press
198 Madison Avenue, New York, NY 10016, United States of America

British Library Cataloguing in Publication Data
Data available

Library of Congress Control Number: 2014949003

ISBN 978–0–19–965139–9

Printed in Great Britain by
Ashford Colour Press Ltd, Gosport, Hampshire

Oxford University Press makes no representation, express or implied, that the
drug dosages in this book are correct. Readers must therefore always check
the product information and clinical procedures with the most up-to-date
published product information and data sheets provided by the manufacturers
and the most recent codes of conduct and safety regulations. The authors and
the publishers do not accept responsibility or legal liability for any errors in the
text or for the misuse or misapplication of material in this work. Except where
otherwise stated, drug dosages and recommendations are for the non-pregnant
adult who is not breast-feeding.

FOREWORD

As medical knowledge expands and technology develops getting access to information in a timely fashion becomes ever more important. This is especially true in specialties such as obstetrics and gynaecology that have both an elective and a significant emergency component.

We all fundamentally practice to achieve the best outcome for all our patients, recognizing the frailties of our ability to keep everything we ever needed to know at our fingertips. The well documented variation in health outcomes, at individual, local, national and international levels is often attributed to the lack of, or inability, to implement best practice.

Simply keeping up to date can be difficult, especially so in the emergency situation. There are a plethora of standards and guidelines available worldwide that through standardization of clinical care aim to improve outcomes. However, access to succinct material in an easy to read and follow algorithm is often difficult to find, especially in the heat of the moment. The authors are to be to be congratulated with this book which I suspect will be a very welcome addition to all our clinics, delivery suites and emergency rooms amongst all professionals who deliver women's healthcare.

David Richmond
President, RCOG

CONTENTS

DETAILED CONTENTS

SECTION 4 Gynaecology emergency presentations 259

CONTRIBUTORS

Nikolaos Burbos
Consultant Gynaecological Oncologist
Norfolk and Norwich University Hospitals NHS
Foundation Trust,
Norwich, UK

Martin J. Cameron
Consultant Obstetrician
Norfolk and Norwich University Hospitals NHS
Foundation Trust,
Norwich, UK

Claudine Domoney
Gynaecology Clinical Effectiveness Lead,
Lead Consultant for Community Gynaecology
and Perineal Services,
Chelsea and Westminster Hospital NHS
Foundation Trust,
London, UK

Stergios Doumouchtsis
Consultant Obstetrician and Gynaecologist,
RCOG Accredited Subspecialist in Urogynaecology,
Honorary Senior Lecturer,
Lead Consultant Urogynaecologist,
Lead Consultant for Childbirth Injury and Pelvic Health
after Childbirth,
Urogynaecology, Female Pelvic Medicine, and
Reconstructive Surgery Unit,
St George's Healthcare NHS Trust, St George's
University of London
London, UK

Tim J. Duncan
Consultant Gynaecological Oncologist,
Department of Obstetrics and Gynaecology,
Norfolk and Norwich University Hospitals NHS
Foundation Trust,
Norwich, UK

Tarek El-Toukhy
Consultant and Honorary Senior Lecturer in
Reproductive Medicine and Surgery,
Guy's and St Thomas' Hospital NHS Foundation Trust,
London, UK

Jo Evans
Consultant in Genitourinary Medicine and HIV,
Norfolk and Norwich University Hospitals NHS
Foundation Trust,
Norwich, UK

David Fraser
Consultant Obstetrician and Gynaecologist,
Norfolk and Norwich University Hospitals NHS
Foundation Trust,
Norwich, UK

Françoise-Hélène D. Harlow
Consultant Obstetrician,
Norfolk and Norwich University Hospitals NHS
Foundation Trust,
Norwich, UK

Clair Jones
Clinical Physiotherapy Specialist, Women's Health,
Norfolk and Norwich University Hospitals NHS
Foundation Trust,
Norwich, UK

Sarah Machin
[work title],
Norfolk and Norwich University Hospitals NHS
Foundation Trust,
Norwich, UK

William Maina
Speciality Doctor, Obstetrics and Gynaecology
Norfolk and Norwich University Hospitals NHS
Foundation Trust,
Norwich, UK

Alastair McKelvey
Consultant Obstetrician, Subspecialist in Maternal-Fetal
Medicine,
Norfolk and Norwich University Hospitals NHS
Foundation Trust,
Norwich, UK

Edward Morris
Consultant in Obstetrics and Gynaecology,
Norfolk and Norwich University Hospitals NHS
Foundation Trust,
Norwich, UK

Sambit Mukhopadhyay
Consultant Obstetrician and Gynaecologist,
Norfolk and Norwich University Hospitals NHS
Foundation Trust,
Norwich, UK

Kate Nash
Locum Consultant in Sexual and Reproductive Health,
Contraception and Sexual Health Service, East Coast
Community Healthcare,
Great Yarmouth and Lowestoft, UK

xiv

Contributors

Joaquin J. Nieto
Consultant Gynaecological Oncologist,
Norfolk and Norwich University Hospitals NHS
Foundation Trust,
Norwich, UK

Daisy Nirmal
Consultant Obstetrician and Gynaecologist,
Norfolk and Norwich University Hospitals NHS
Foundation Trust,
Norwich, UK

Richards A. Onifade
Norfolk and Norwich University Hospitals NHS
Foundation Trust,
Norwich, UK,

Thilina Palihawadana
Clinical Fellow,
Norfolk and Norwich University Hospitals NHS
Foundation Trust,
Norwich, UK

Edward Prosser-Snelling
Norfolk and Norwich University Hospitals NHS
Foundation Trust,
Norwich, UK

Gautam Raje
Consultant Obstetrician and Gynaecologist,
Norfolk and Norwich University Hospitals NHS
Foundation Trust,
Norwich, UK

Vladimir Revicky
Specialty Registrar in Obstetrics and Gynaecology,
Cambridge University Hospitals NHS Foundation Trust,
Cambridge, UK

Richard Smith
Consultant Obstetrician, Subspecialist in Fetal Medicine,
Clinical Tutor,

Norfolk and Norwich University Hospitals NHS
Foundation Trust,
Norwich, UK

Katharine P. Stanley
Consultant Obstetrician and Gynaecologist,
Norfolk and Norwich University Hospitals NHS
Foundation Trust,
Norwich, UK

Medha Sule
Consultant Gynaecologist and Obstetrician,
Honorary Senior lecturer, Clinical Skills Coordinator,
Norfolk and Norwich University Hospitals NHS
Foundation Trust,
Norwich, UK

Vikram S. Talaulikar
Clinical Research Fellow,
Department of Obstetrics and Gynaecology,
St. George's Hospital and University of London,
London, UK

Eman Toeima
Specialty Doctor,
Norfolk and Norwich University Hospitals NHS
Foundation Trust,
Norwich, UK

Hilary Turnbull
Norfolk and Norwich University Hospitals NHS
Foundation Trust,
Norwich, UK

Richard C. Warren
Consultant Obstetrician and Gynaecologist,
Norfolk and Norwich University Hospitals NHS
Foundation Trust,
Norwich, UK

SYMBOLS AND ABBREVIATIONS

α	alpha
β	beta
°	degree
°C	degree Celsius
≥	equal to or greater than
≤	equal to or less than
>	greater than
λ	lambda
<	less than
%	per cent
£	pound sterling
®	registered trademark
±	with or without
ABG	arterial blood gas
ACE	angiotensin-converting enzyme
A & E	accident and emergency
AFC	antral follicle count
AFI	amniotic fluid index
AFP	alpha-fetoprotein
AMH	anti-Müllerian hormone
APH	antepartum haemorrhage
APS	antiphospholipid syndrome
APTT	activated partial thromboplastin time
ARDS	adult/acute respiratory distress syndrome
ARM	artificial rupture of fetal membranes
ASB	asymptomatic bacteriuria
BAC	birth after Caesarean
bd	twice daily
β-hCG	beta-human chorionic gonadotrophin
BMI	body mass index
BNF	British National Formulary
BP	blood pressure
BPD	bronchopulmonary dysplasia
bpm	beat per minute
BSO	bilateral salpingo-oophorectomy
BV	bacterial vaginosis
CCT	controlled cord contraction
CEA	carcinoembryonic antigen
CHD	congenital heart disease
CI	confidential interval
CIN	cervical intraepithelial neoplasia
cm	centimetre
CMV	cytomegalovirus
CMW	community midwife
CNS	central nervous system
COC	combined oral contraceptive
COCP	combined oral contraceptive pill
COX	cyclo-oxygenase
CPR	cardiopulmonary resuscitation
CRP	C-reactive protein
C/S	Caesarean section
CT	computed tomography
CTG	cardiotocography
CTPA	computed tomography pulmonary angiography
Cu IUD	copper intrauterine device
CVS	chorionic villus sampling
CXR	chest X-ray
3-D	three-dimensional
DES	diethylstilboestrol

DIC	disseminated intravascular coagulation		FMH	fetomaternal haemorrhage
dL	decilitre		FSH	follicle-stimulating hormone
DM	diabetes mellitus		g	gram
DNA	deoxyribonucleic acid		GBS	group B Streptococcus
DRSP	daily record of severity of problems		GDM	gestational diabetes mellitus
DSP	diastasis symphysis pubis		GI	gastrointestinal
DVT	deep venous thrombosis		GnRH	gonadotrophin-releasing hormone
D/W	discuss with		GnRH-a	gonadotrophin-releasing hormone agonist
EAS	external anal sphincter		GP	general practitioner
EBV	Epstein–Barr virus		GS	gestational sac
EC	emergency contraception		G & S	group and save
ECG	electrocardiogram		GTD	gestational trophoblastic disease
ECT	electroconvulsive therapy		GTN	gestational trophoblastic neoplasia
ECV	external cephalic version		GTT	glucose tolerance test
EFM	electronic fetal monitoring		GUM	genitourinary medicine
EFW	estimated fetal weight		Gy	gray
EPAU	Early Pregnancy Advisory Unit		h	hour
ERCS	elective repeat Caesarean		Hb	haemoglobin
ERT	(o)estrogen-only replacement therapy		HBeAg	hepatitis B virus e-antigen
ESR	erythrocyte sedimentation rate		HBIG	hepatitis B-specific immune globulin
ET	endometrial thickness		HBV	hepatitis B virus
ETT	epithelioid trophoblastic tumour		hCG	human chorionic gonadotrophin
EUA	examination under anaesthesia		HDFN	haemolytic disease of the fetus and newborn
FAI	free androgen index			
FBC	full blood count		HDU	high dependency unit
FBS	fetal blood sampling		HELLP	haemolysis, elevated liver enzymes, and low platelets
FDA	Food and Drug Administration			
FEV1	forced expiratory volume in 1 second		HIV	human immunodeficiency virus
FHR	fetal heart rate		HMB	heavy menstrual bleeding
FIGO	International Federation of Gynecologists and Obstetricians (Fédération Internationale de Gynécologie et d'Obstétrique)		H/O	history of
			HPLC	high-performance liquid chromatography
			HPV	human papillomavirus
			HRT	hormone replacement therapy
fL	femtolitre		HVS	high vaginal swab

IAS	internal anal sphincter	LNG-IUS	levonorgestrel-releasing intrauterine system
IBS	irritable bowel syndrome	LSCS	lower section Caesarean section
ICSI	intracytoplasmic sperm injection	m	metre
Ig	immunoglobulin	MCA	middle cerebral artery
IM	intramuscular	M, C, & S	microscopy, culture, and sensitivity
IOL	induction of labour	MCV	mean corpuscular volume
ITU	intensive treatment unit	MDMA	3,4-methylenedioxymethamphetamine
IU	international unit	mg	milligram
IUCD	intrauterine contraceptive device	MgSO4	magnesium sulfate
IUFD	intrauterine fetal death	MHRA	Medical and Healthcare products Regulatory Agency
IUGR	intrauterine growth restriction	MHz	megahertz
IUI	intrauterine insemination	min	minute
IUS	intrauterine system	mIU	milli international unit
IUT	in utero blood transfusion	mL	millilitre
IV	intravenous	mm	millimetre
IVC	inferior vena cava	mmHg	millimetre of mercury
IVF	in vitro fertilization	mmol	millimole
IVH	intraventricular haemorrhage	MMR	mumps, measles, and rubella
IVI	intravenous infusion	MRI	magnetic resonance imaging
J	joule	MS	multiple sclerosis
JVP	jugular venous pressure	MSU	midstream urine sample
kg	kilogram	NEC	necrotizing enterocolitis
kU	kilounit	NGT	nasogastric tube
L	litre	NHS	National Health Service
LARC	long-acting reversible contraception	NHSLA	National Health Service Litigation Authority
LBP	low back pain	NICE	National Institute for Health and Clinical Excellence
LDH	lactate dehydrogenase		
LFT	liver function test	NICU	neonatal intensive care unit
LH	luteinizing hormone	nmol	nanomole
LLETZ	large loop excision of the transformation zone	NPSA	National Patient Safety Agency
LMP	last menstrual period	NSAID	non-steroidal anti-inflammatory drug
LMWH	low-molecular-weight heparin		
LNG	levonorgestrel		

NTD	neural tube defect
OAB	overactive bladder
od	once daily
OHSS	ovarian hyperstimulation syndrome
PAPP-A	pregnancy-associated plasma protein A
PC	personal computer
PCOS	polycystic ovarian syndrome
PCR	polymerase chain reaction
PDA	patent ductus arteriosus
PDD	premenstrual dysphoric disorder
PDS	polydioxanone
PE	pulmonary embolism
PEA	pulseless electrical activity
PEFR	peak expiratory flow rate
PET	positron emission tomography
PFME	pelvic floor muscle exercise
PFMT	pelvic floor muscle training
pg	picogram
PG	prostaglandin
PGP	pelvic girdle pain
PID	pelvic inflammatory disease
PMB	post-menopausal bleeding
pmol	picomole
PMS	premenstrual syndrome
PO	orally
POP-Q	pelvic organ prolapse quantification
PPH	post-partum haemorrhage
PPROM	preterm prelabour rupture of the membranes
prn	as required
PR	per rectum
PRL	prolactin
PSTT	placental site trophoblastic tumour
PTU	propylthiouracil

PUPP	pruritic urticarial papules and plaques of pregnancy
PV	per vagina
RCOG	Royal College of Obstetricians and Gynaecologists
RDS	respiratory distress syndrome
RFM	reduced fetal movement
Rh	rhesus
RIF	right iliac fossa
RMI	risk of malignancy index
ROM	rupture of membranes
RR	relative risk
s	second
SARC	Sexual Assault Referral Centre
SC	subcutaneous
SFH	symphysis fundal height
SGA	small for gestational age
SHBG	sex hormone-binding globulin
SLE	systemic lupus erythematosus
SNRI	serotonin-noradrenaline reuptake inhibitor
SPD	symphysis pubis dysfunction
SROM	spontaneous rupture of the amniotic membranes
SSRI	selective serotonin reuptake inhibitor
STD	sexually transmitted disease
STI	sexually transmitted infection
T4	thyroxine
TAH	total abdominal hysterectomy
TAUS	transabdominal ultrasonography
tds	three times daily
TED	thromboembolism deterrent
TENS	transcutaneous electrical nerve stimulation
TFT	thyroid function test
TOP	termination of pregnancy

TORCH	toxoplasmosis, rubella, cytomegalovirus, hepatitis	UPD	uniparental disomy
		UPI	uteroplacental insufficiency
TPN	total parenteral nutrition	UPSI	unprotected sexual intercourse
TRAb	thyroid-stimulating hormone receptor-stimulating antibodies	US	United States
		USS	ultrasound scan
TSH	thyroid-stimulating hormone	UTI	urinary tract infection
TTTS	twin-twin transfusion syndrome	VBAC	vaginal birth after Caesarean section
TV	transvaginal; Trichomonas vaginalis	VEGF	vascular endothelial growth factor
TVS	transvaginal ultrasound scan	VF	ventricular fibrillation
TVUS	transvaginal ultrasonography	VIN	vulval intraepithelial neoplasia
U	unit	V/Q	ventilation/perfusion
UAE	uterine artery embolization	vs	versus
U + Es	urea and electrolytes	VT	ventricular tachycardia
UI	urinary incontinence	VTE	venous thromboembolism
UK	United Kingdom	WBC	white blood cell
UKMEC	United Kingdom Medical Eligibility Criteria	WHO	World Health Organization
UPA	ulipristal acetate	YS	yolk sac

SECTION 1

Non-urgent obstetrics

Diagnosis of pregnancy

Key learning points

Methods of diagnosis of pregnancy

Role of radioimmunoassay

Role of ultrasound scan.

Introduction

Pregnancy can be diagnosed by a combination of history/physical examination, laboratory tests, or ultrasound examination.

History

- Amenorrhoea
- Menstrual history
- Date of onset of last menstrual bleeding (LMP)
- Duration of menstrual bleeding
- Frequency/irregularity of menstrual bleeding
- Use of contraception
- Atypical last menstrual bleeding
- Use of *in vitro* fertilization (IVF) techniques.

Physical examination

- Breast changes (darkening of nipples)
- Blue discoloration of the cervix and vagina (Chadwick's sign)
- Softening of the cervix (Goodell's sign)
- Enlarged cervix and softening—ability to approximate fingers in the vagina from behind and in front on the abdomen across the isthmus (Hegar's sign)
- Softening of the uterus (Ladin's sign)
- Enlarged uterus on bimanual examination.

Laboratory tests

Beta-human chorionic gonadotrophin (beta-hCG):

- hCG is a glycoprotein composed of alpha and beta subunits
- The alpha subunit is similar to the alpha subunit of FSH, LH, and thyrotropin
- hCG is present in the maternal circulation as either an intact dimer, alpha or beta subunit, or beta core fragment
- The beta core fragment emerges as the predominant form in the **fifth week** after conception
- The beta subunit core fragment is primarily detected by pregnancy tests in urine samples
- Most current urinary pregnancy tests have sensitivity to approximately 25 mIU/mL.

There are four types of immunoassays.

- Radioimmunoassay
  - Sensitivity—5 mIU/mL
  - Gestational age when first positive—3–4 weeks
- Immunoradiometric assay
  - Sensitivity—150 mIU/mL
  - Gestational age when first positive—4 weeks

- Enzyme-linked immunosorbent assay
  - Sensitivity—25 mIU/mL
  - Gestational age when first positive—3.5 weeks
- Fluoroimmunoassay
  - Sensitivity—1 mIU/mL
  - Gestational age when first positive—3.5 weeks.

Serial hCG monitoring:

- At 4 weeks' gestation, hCG doubling times are approximately 2.2 days
- By 9 weeks' gestation, hCG doubling times are approximately 3.5 days
- hCG levels peak at 10–12 weeks' gestation
- Failure to achieve the projected rate of rise of hCG may suggest an ectopic pregnancy, non-viable pregnancy, or spontaneous abortion.

Ultrasonography

- Transvaginal ultrasonography (TVUS) with frequency of 5–8 MHz
- Transabdominal ultrasonography (TAUS) with frequency of 3–5 MHz
- TVUS detect signs of intrauterine pregnancy approximately 1 week earlier than TAUS
- TVUS is the most accurate means of confirming intrauterine pregnancy and gestational age during the early first trimester
- If hCG levels are >1000–1500 mIU/mL, pregnancy structures should be identifiable inside the uterus
- If no intrauterine pregnancy structures on TVUS and hCG >1000–1500 mIU/mL, ectopic pregnancy is a possible diagnosis.

Structures of pregnancy are identified by TVUS in a chronologic order:

- Gestational sac (GS) by 4–5 weeks of gestation
- Double-decidual sign (GS surrounded by the thickened deciduas) by 5.5–6 weeks
- Yolk sac (YS) by 4–5 weeks—diagnosis of intrauterine pregnancy
- Fetal pole by 5–6 weeks
- Fetal heart by 5–6 weeks.

Further reading

Royal College of Obstetricians and Gynaecologists (2006). *The management of early pregnancy loss.* Green-top guideline No. 25. Available at: <http://www.rcog.org.uk/files/rcog-corp/uploaded-files/GT25ManagementofEarlyPregnancyLoss2006.pdf>.

Care pathway for the diagnosis of pregnancy

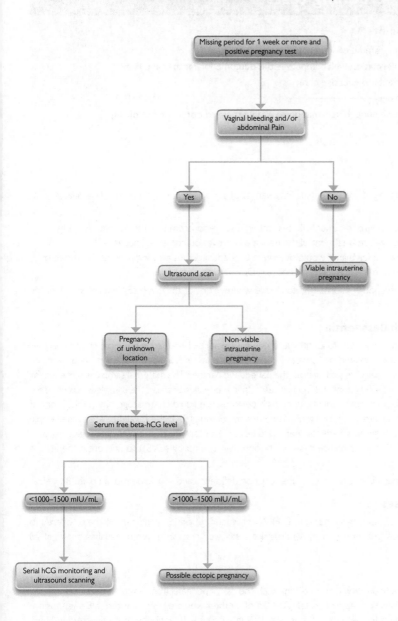

Antenatal screening tests

Key learning points

Part of a national programme of screening

Tests can provide information which improves the outcome for mother and baby

Tests may allow patients to exercise choice

Tests may create anxiety

Patients should receive enough information to enable them to opt in, or out of, any screening tests.

Introduction

Pregnant women should be offered screening for a variety of conditions during pregnancy. Potential benefits include:

- Identifying a condition where treatment of the mother improves outcome for the neonate (e.g. HIV)
- Identifying a condition where treatment of the neonate improves outcome (e.g. hepatitis B)
- Identifying a condition earlier than it would otherwise be identified, thus allowing patients the choice of whether to continue with the pregnancy or not (e.g. Down's syndrome).

Patients should be given enough information to decide whether or not they wish to have any, or all, of the screening tests.

Sickle cell and thalassaemia

Haemoglobinopathy screening aims to identify fetuses who are at risk because both the patient and partner are carriers. It should be completed by 10 weeks of pregnancy. It involves a blood test from the patient and a 'family of origin questionnaire' regarding both the patient and partner. The maternal sample is screened for thalassaemia, using a full blood count (FBC) in all cases. In low prevalence areas, the sample is screened for sickle cell and other haemoglobin variants, using high-performance liquid chromatography (HPLC), only if the patient or partner is from a high-risk group (deemed by ancestry). In high-prevalence areas, the sample is screened using HPLC regardless. Patients deemed to be at risk of carrying a fetus with haemoglobinopathy are offered invasive testing (i.e. amniocentesis or chorionic villus sampling (CVS)) to find out if the fetus is affected.

FBC also screens for anaemia due to other causes, e.g. iron deficiency, and should be repeated at 28 weeks.

Infectious diseases

This includes screening at booking for hepatitis B, HIV, syphilis, and rubella. Screening should be re-offered to those in high-risk groups (e.g. intravenous (IV) drug users, sex workers, those with bisexual partners) at 28 weeks of pregnancy.

Hepatitis B

The incidence in the UK population is around 1 in 1000. The risk of perinatal transmission is dependent on the status of the maternal infection. Approximately 70–90% of mothers who are HBV e antigen (HBeAg)-positive will transmit the infection to the neonate, but only 10% in women with antibody to e antigen (anti-HBe). Vaccination of the neonate within 24 h of delivery and at 1, 2, and 12 months is effective in preventing vertical transmission. In neonates born to patients with a higher risk of transmission, the addition of hepatitis B-specific immune globulin (HBIG) can reduce the risk further.

Human immunodeficiency virus (HIV)

The incidence of previously undiagnosed HIV in pregnancy is around 1 in 1000 in the UK. The precise management of patients who are infected will depend on factors such as the viral load, but treatment with antiretroviral therapy, delivery by Caesarean section (C/S) in appropriate cases, and avoidance of breastfeeding greatly reduce the risk of vertical transmission from 15–25% to 1% or less. Screening for other sexually transmitted infections (STIs) should be offered.

Syphilis

The incidence of syphilis in pregnancy is very low and, therefore, difficult to estimate but is probably in the order of 1 in 10 000 pregnancies in the UK. The risk of vertical transmission is high, ranging from 70 to 100% in primary syphilis, 40% in early latent syphilis, and 10% in late latent syphilis. Maternal syphilis infection can result in a range of adverse outcomes, including late miscarriage, stillbirth, hydrops, and low birthweight. If left untreated, congenital syphilis can result in physical and neurological impairments, affecting the child's bones, teeth, vision, and hearing. Early recognition and treatment (usually with penicillin) can prevent these adverse outcomes.

Rubella

Screening for rubella is different to the preceding three tests, as the test is not performed to screen for infection during pregnancy, but to identify patients who are not immune (about 3% of the childbearing population in the UK). Patients who are not immune can be advised to avoid contact with anyone suffering from rubella and offered the mumps, measles, and rubella (MMR) vaccine in the post-natal period to eliminate the risk of congenital rubella in future pregnancies.

Blood group and antibodies

Fifteen per cent of patients are rhesus D-negative. These patients are offered prophylactic anti-D injections later in pregnancy to reduce the chance of sensitization, and, therefore, reduce the chances of haemolytic disease of the newborn in the current or future pregnancies.

The test will also identify a small number of women who already have antibodies present against red blood cell antigens. This group of women will require increased surveillance with antibody monitoring and possibly ultrasound to look for signs of fetal anaemia. The antibody screen is repeated at 28 weeks.

Down's syndrome

About one in 800 pregnancies would result in a live born child with Down's syndrome without screening. Although the incidence becomes greater as maternal age advances, the majority of pregnancies occur in women under 30 years of age, so age alone is not a good screening tool.

The combined test is performed between 11 weeks 2 days and 14 weeks 1 day of pregnancy. This combines the results of ultrasound and biochemical findings. The ultrasound findings are the crown rump length and the nuchal translucency measurement. The biochemical markers are pregnancy-associated plasma protein A (PAPP-A) and free beta-human chorionic gonadotrophin (β-hCG). This combination has a screen positive rate of 3% for an 85% detection rate (sensitivity).

Those who book too late for a combined test, or those in whom it is not possible to measure the nuchal translucency, should be offered the quadruple test. This is a biochemical test (although it relies on accurate ultrasound dating) and can be performed between 14 weeks 2 days and 20 weeks 0 days of pregnancy. It has a screen positive rate of around 4% for an 80% detection rate.

Patients identified as at higher risk (greater than 1 in 150) will be offered a diagnostic test (CVS or amniocentesis).

Fetal anomaly scan

This is performed between 18 weeks 0 days and 20 weeks 6 days to look for structural abnormalities in the fetus. Recently, the national screening committee has identified 11 conditions, which the scan can be expected to screen for (see Key information). The detection rate of different conditions varies greatly, for instance, anencephaly should be detected in at least 98% of cases, whereas serious cardiac abnormalities will have a minimum detection rate of only 50%. Patients who are found to have a fetus with a structural problem will usually be referred to a fetal medicine specialist.

Communication of results

Most patients will be reassured by normal or low-risk results of their test. Those who have abnormal results will be referred through the appropriate specialist. The neonatal team is informed of any results that are of relevance, e.g. a structural abnormality in the fetus that may require immediate neonatal care or a fetus requiring vaccination for hepatitis B.

Further reading

UK Screening Portal. UK National Screening Committee. Available at: <http://www.screening.nhs.uk/uknsc>.

Key information for the 11 conditions for which the UK National Screening Committee recommends should be screened at the fetal anomaly scan, and their minimum detection rates

Condition	Chance of being seen (%)
Anencephaly	98
Open spina bifida	90
Cleft	75
Diaphragmatic hernia	60
Gastroschisis	98
Exomphalos	80
Serious cardiac abnormalities	50
Bilateral renal agenesis	84
Lethal skeletal dysplasia	60
Edwards' syndrome (trisomy 18)	95
Patau's syndrome (trisomy 13)	95

Available at: <http://www.fetalanomaly.screening.nhs.uk/getdata. php?id=11218>. This information was originally developed by the UK National Screening Committee/NHS Screening Programmes (www.screening.nhs.uk) and is used under the Open Government Licence v2.0: <http://www.nationalarchives.gov.uk/ doc/open-government-licence/version/2/>

Infections and vaccinations in pregnancy

Key learning points

Fetal and perinatal implications of maternal infection during pregnancy differ according to the causative organism and stage of gestation

Reducing risk from infection can be attained through prophylactic vaccination or assessing inherent immunity

Management of infected pregnancies includes maternal and, in some cases, fetal testing.

Introduction

Most of the infections in pregnancy are caused by genital tract flora, and their effects on the mother and fetus depend on the gestation, underlying maternal condition, as well as inoculum and virulence of the offending organism.

Fetal and maternal effects

Fetus

Some infections in the first trimester of pregnancy can have teratogenic effects and cause defective organogenesis in the embryo, e.g. rubella. If the fetus is affected in the second or third trimester, depending on the type of infection, there can be profound effects on various organ systems such as nervous system, blood, circulatory system, etc. Infection can also lead to stillbirth, preterm deliveries, fetal intrauterine growth restriction (IUGR), and neonatal infection. Severe infections may sometimes result in long-term handicap and neurological sequelae in newborns.

Mother

It is suggested that pregnancy is an immunosuppressive state, and infections in the mother may vary in severity from asymptomatic bacteriuria to severe pyelonephritis and life-threatening sepsis. Some infections, such as vaginal candidiasis and urinary tract infections (UTIs), are encountered more frequently in pregnant women while others, such as influenza, chickenpox, and hepatitis E, tend to run a more severe course in pregnancy in comparison to non-pregnant women.

Diagnosis and screening

Screening for evidence of infection prior to, or early in, pregnancy is invaluable for ascertaining the risk of perinatal injury as a consequence of exposure after conception. In the UK, screening is recommended for hepatitis B, HIV, rubella, and syphilis early in pregnancy with a single blood sample, as well as asymptomatic bacteriuria (ASB) with a urine sample. There is currently no clear evidence of benefit from screening for other infections. For screening for group B Streptococcus (GBS), cytomegalovirus (CMV), and toxoplasmosis, each case should be considered on an individual basis. For women at high risk for HIV, it is important to repeat the HIV test in the third trimester. A negative test at booking can be falsely reassuring, and seroconversion may have occurred during pregnancy.

Diagnosis relies on either (1) isolating or detecting the infectious organism, e.g. CMV, malaria, or (2) documenting seroconversion with acquisition of specific antibodies IgM or rise in IgG titre on two consecutive samples 2–4 weeks apart, e.g. toxoplasmosis or rubella.

Primary prevention

Measures to avoid toxoplasmosis infection include thorough hand washing, cooking raw meats, and avoiding contact with cat litter and soil. Prevention of listeriosis involves avoiding eating unpasteurized dairy products or pâté and washing salads thoroughly. Pregnant women should be encouraged to avoid travel to areas where certain diseases are endemic, e.g. toxoplasmosis or malaria.

Vaccinations

Ideally, women should be immunized prior to conception, but there are a few situations where immunization of a pregnant woman is indicated. Live attenuated vaccines, such as rubella, polio, or MMR, are usually contraindicated due to the risk of fetal infection; however, passive immunization with specific human immunoglobulin or tetanus toxoid is safe. Women planning a family should ensure immunity against rubella. Live varicella vaccines are available pre-pregnancy, and zoster immunoglobulin should be given to pregnant women non-immune to varicella and up to 10 days following exposure. Women who are hepatitis B surface antigen-negative, but considered at high risk, should be offered hepatitis B vaccination in pregnancy. Influenza vaccination (inactivated) may be considered and is deemed safe throughout pregnancy. Based on recent experience of H5N1 influenza and its increased severity in pregnant women, all women should be offered the seasonal vaccine which will give protection to the most common circulating strains. Neonatal infection can be prevented in some cases by passive immunization of the newborn, e.g. chickenpox. Vaccination for travel should be considered on an individual basis and the small risk from vaccine compared with the risk from contracting the disease.

There are four types of vaccines:

- Toxoids—produced by organisms
- Inactivated organisms—generally regarded as safe to administer to pregnant women after the first trimester
- Live attenuated vaccines—generally avoided in pregnancy as they may cause infection in the fetus or cause congenital abnormalities
- Immune globulin preparations—pregnancy per se is not a contraindication to immunoglobulins (passive immunization)
- DNA recombinant vaccines—safe to administer in pregnancy.

Management of infections

Once a viral infection is established, little can be done to change its course. There must be careful follow-up of the mother, and the infant must be monitored through early childhood for evidence of the expanded infection syndrome. If the pregnant woman is susceptible and at risk due to exposure, the morbidity and mortality from both maternal and fetal infection must be assessed. For example, tetanus has high maternal mortality and morbidity rates, and risk of neonatal tetanus. Tetanus toxoid is indicated routinely for susceptible pregnant women. Sepsis-related maternal morbidity and mortality are a significant problem, and the management of sepsis during pregnancy can be challenging due to the effect of maternal physiologic changes on fetal vulnerability and the effect of the fetus on maternal status throughout the pregnancy. Early detection, accurate diagnosis, and aggressive appropriate treatment strategies (fluids, antimicrobials, immunoglobulins, supportive therapies) may significantly improve outcomes.

Rubella

The major risk to the fetus from rubella infection exists in the first 12 weeks of pregnancy. The risk is diminished between 13 and 16 weeks, and very little risk remains after 16 weeks.

Fetal defects include ocular defects (cataracts, glaucoma, microphthalmia), heart defects (patent ductus arteriosus (PDA)), sensorineural hearing loss, and mental retardation. Maternal infection is symptomatic in 50–70% in the form of rash, arthritis, and lymphadenopathy. Incubation period is 14–21 days, and infectivity is 7 days before and after rash. Prevention relies on rubella/MMR vaccination before conception.

Cytomegalovirus

The fetus is at risk in all trimesters of pregnancy. Defects include microcephaly, hepatosplenomegaly, jaundice, IUGR, thrombocytopenia, chorioretinitis, and intracranial calcifications. Maternal infection is usually subclinical. Risk of fetal defects is about 4% with maternal infection.

Varicella

Although varicella infection can pose risk in all trimesters, the highest fetal risk exists between 13 and 20 weeks. It may result in hypoplasia or aplasia of single limbs, with skin cicatrization, deafness, psychomotor retardation, and ocular abnormalities. The incubation period is 14–21 days, and infectivity is from 1 day prior up to 6 days after the disappearance of the rash. Oral aciclovir reduces the duration of symptoms if given within 24 h of the rash appearing. Varicella in pregnancy is often more severe and may be life-threatening due to pneumonia, hepatitis, or encephalitis. If a woman has an exposure without history of previous infection, serum should be tested for IgG antibodies. If antibodies are positive within 10 days of contact, assume immunity. If not positive, varicella immunoglobulin should be given as soon as possible. Neonatal varicella may be seen in mothers infected in the last 4 weeks of pregnancy. These babies should receive immunoglobulins as soon as possible.

Parvovirus B19

Maternal infection presents with 'slapped cheek' rash (erythema infectiosum), fever, and arthralgia. The incubation period is 4–20 days. Fetal risks include miscarriage, hydrops fetalis, anaemia, and fetal death. Testing is based on detection of parvovirus B19 IgM and IgG antibodies. Management in affected pregnancies (in specialist fetal medicine unit) includes serial ultrasound scans, Doppler measurements of middle cerebral artery blood flow, and blood transfusions *in utero* to treat fetal anaemia.

Toxoplasmosis

Maternal infection is asymptomatic in about 80%. Symptoms include fever and lymphadenopathy. Measures to avoid toxoplasmosis infection include thorough hand washing, cooking raw meats, and avoiding contact with cat litter and soil. Major risk of transmission of infection to the fetus lies in the third trimester (65%); however, the risk of anomalies is <10%. In contrast, although 15–20% of fetuses may be affected in the first trimester, there is a high risk (75%) of fetal anomalies. Defects include chorioretinitis, microcephaly, hydrocephalus, intracranial calcifications, and mental retardation. Starting spiramycin on diagnosis may decrease the risk of fetal infection. If fetal infection occurs, combination anti-toxoplasmosis therapy (pyrimethamine/sulfadiazine) is used.

Listeriosis

Women may be asymptomatic or have a febrile flu-like illness. Severe infection may lead to ARDS (acute respiratory distress syndrome). Women should be advised to avoid high-risk foods, unpasteurized dairy products, and pâté. Listeriosis may cause miscarriage, preterm labour, and meconium staining. Prolonged parenteral antibiotics (ampicillin and gentamicin) should be given until 1 week after fever subsides.

Further reading

National Institute for Health and Clinical Excellence (2008). *Antenatal care: routine care for the healthy pregnant woman.* NICE clinical guideline 62. Available at: <http://www.nice.org.uk/nicemedia/pdf/CG062NICEguideline.pdf>.

Algorithm for the management of toxoplasmosis in pregnancy

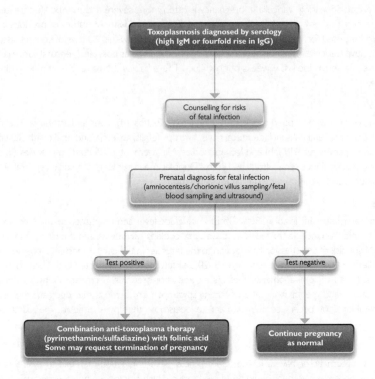

Toxoplasmosis diagnosed by serology
(high IgM or fourfold rise in IgG)

Counselling for risks
of fetal infection

Prenatal diagnosis for fetal infection
(amniocentesis/chorionic villus sampling/fetal
blood sampling and ultrasound)

Test positive

Test negative

Combination anti-toxoplasma therapy
(pyrimethamine/sulfadiazine) with folinic acid
Some may request termination of pregnancy

Continue pregnancy
as normal

Algorithm for the management of chickenpox in pregnancy

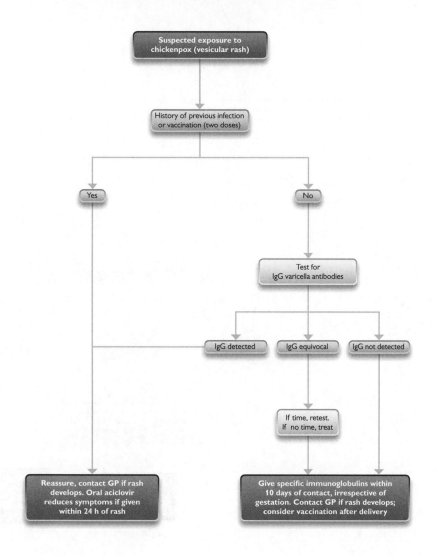

Suspected exposure to chickenpox (vesicular rash)

History of previous infection or vaccination (two doses)

Yes

No

Test for IgG varicella antibodies

IgG detected

IgG equivocal

IgG not detected

If time, retest. If no time, treat

Reassure, contact GP if rash develops. Oral aciclovir reduces symptoms if given within 24 h of rash

Give specific immunoglobulins within 10 days of contact, irrespective of gestation. Contact GP if rash develops; consider vaccination after delivery

Algorithm for the management of rubella in pregnancy

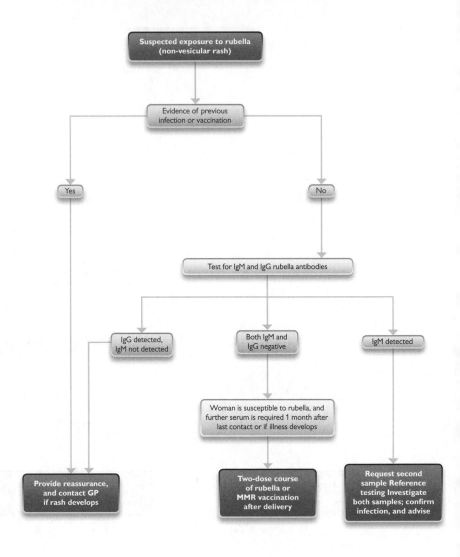

Suspected exposure to rubella (non-vesicular rash)

Evidence of previous infection or vaccination

Yes

No

Test for IgM and IgG rubella antibodies

IgG detected, IgM not detected

Both IgM and IgG negative

IgM detected

Woman is susceptible to rubella, and further serum is required 1 month after last contact or if illness develops

Provide reassurance, and contact GP if rash develops

Two-dose course of rubella or MMR vaccination after delivery

Request second sample Reference testing Investigate both samples; confirm infection, and advise

Medications in pregnancy

Key learning points

Women taking medication should have indications and doses reviewed

Caution should be exercised when prescribing any medication during pregnancy

Report adverse outcomes following prescribing.

Introduction

When considering prescribing a drug to a pregnant woman, several factors must be considered:

- Gestational age
- Route of administration
- Absorption rate
- Effect of pregnancy on absorption/elimination and distribution
- Whether drug crosses the placenta and/or is secreted into breast milk
- Dose and duration of therapy
- Potential harm to fetus/infant from drug
- Potential harm to mother if drug withheld
- Are safer alternatives available?

Ultimately, you need to determine if benefits of the drug outweigh its risks.

Drug pharmacokinetics and pregnancy

Although gastric emptying time is reduced in pregnancy, this has little effect on drug absorption. There is, however, increased absorption of bronchodilators by the lungs.

Change in plasma volume, body fat, and albumin levels can affect drug distribution.

As glomerular filtration rate increases by 50% in pregnancy, there is increased renal clearance of drugs.

All medications are classified by the United States Food and Drug Administration in regard to their risk in pregnancy (see Table 1). This can aid decisions to start, continue, discontinue, or alter medication in pregnancy but should not be relied on exclusively, as each case should be analysed separately and risks vs benefits calculated.

Management

Ideally, review women on medication prior to pregnancy so these can be reviewed, optimized, and/or altered prior to pregnancy as well as to give the woman time to become stable on any new medication.

Table 1 United States Food and Drug Administration classifications

FDA category	Pregnancy category definition
A	**Controlled studies showed no risk to humans.** No studies in pregnant women have shown an increased risk of fetal anomalies
B	**No evidence of risk in humans.** Animal studies have shown no risk to the fetus; however, no good studies in pregnant women **or** animal studies have shown an adverse effect, but this has not been confirmed in human studies
C	**Risks cannot be ruled out in humans.** Animal studies have shown an adverse effect, and no studies in pregnant women **or** no studies in animals or pregnant women
D	**Clear evidence of risk in humans.** Adequate studies in pregnant women have identified risk, but these may be outweighed by benefits of therapy
X	**Drugs contraindicated in human pregnancy.** Studies have shown risk of fetal abnormalities. Drugs contraindicated in pregnancy and in women who may become pregnant

Reproduced with permission from U.S. Food and Drug Administration.

Discourage women from simply stopping their medications in pregnancy, as risks of this may outweigh any potential benefit.

Only prescribe drugs to pregnant women when the indications are clear.

When possible, use drugs which have been well trialled in pregnancy.

Use the smallest effective dose for the shortest possible time.

If necessary, consult with other specialists prior to commencing, altering, or ceasing medication.

Report adverse effects to external agencies such as the National Teratology Service (UK).
Consider additional scans if a patient is on drugs in class C, D, or X.

Further reading

Buhimschi CS and Weiner CP (2009). Medications in pregnancy and lactation: Part 1. Teratology. *Obstetrics and Gynecology*, **113**, 166–88.

Buhimschi CS and Weiner CP (2009). Medications in pregnancy and lactation: Part 2. Drugs with minimal or unknown human teratogenic effect. *Obstetrics and Gynecology*, **113**, 417–32.

Care pathway for medications in pregnancy

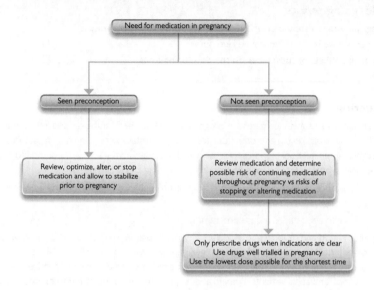

Substance misuse in pregnancy

Key learning points
All pregnant women should be asked about alcohol or substance misuse
Multi-agency care is key to improved outcomes
Consider the effects of substances on the developing fetus.

Introduction
The incidence of most substance misuse in pregnancy is unknown. It can be divided into non-illicit (e.g. alcohol) and illicit (cannabis, heroin and other opiates, cocaine, ecstasy, ketamine, etc.) substances. All pregnant women at their antenatal booking visit should be asked questions about alcohol consumption and use of illicit drugs to identify women who may need enhanced care during and after pregnancy.

NICE clinical guidance makes several recommendations to enhance care for pregnant women who misuse substances, including:

1. Offer referral to a substance misuse programme
2. Offer information and support about additional services available to her (e.g. drugs and alcohol support services), potential effects of the drug(s) on her baby and what to expect when the baby is born (medical care required, where the baby will be cared for, involvement of social services), and help with transport to attend appointments. Remind about appointments, using various methods (e.g. texting)
3. Work with social care professionals to provide supportive and coordinated care, which can address a woman's fears about children's services involvement and the potential removal of her child, and address her feelings of guilt about her substance misuse and the potential effects on her baby.

Alcohol misuse
Several questionnaire tools are available for screening—a very simple tool is the CAGE questionnaire which comprises discriminating questions where two affirmative questions strongly predicts alcoholism.

Alcohol addiction
- Women drinking >6 U of alcohol daily are at greatest risk of fetal alcohol syndrome
- Incidence varies between 0.33 and 1.9/1000 births
- Fetal alcohol syndrome is associated with growth restriction, hand and facial deformities, and intellectual impairment
- More than two 'glasses' of alcohol a day may lead to fetal alcohol effects—problems with learning speech, language, attention span, and hyperactivity.

Specific pregnancy issues
- Consultant-led care with specialist team
- Detailed anomaly scan, followed by serial growth scans
- Screen for liver disease and clotting disorders; consider other health issues (e.g. oesophageal varices, blood-borne infections).

Heroin addiction
Colloquially: boy, brown, china white, dragon, gear, H, horse, junk, skag, smack.
- Heroin is a class A drug. Smoked, sniffed, or injected as a solution. Not teratogenic
- 0.1% of 16–24 year olds report having used heroin in the last year in the 2010–11 British Crime Survey
- 0.4% of 16–24 year olds report use of methadone in the last year.

- Pregnancy associations are preterm delivery, fetal growth restriction, antepartum haemorrhage (APH), and multiple pregnancy
- Replacement therapy: methadone or buprenorphine (Subutex®).

Specific pregnancy issues

- The aim is to 'stabilize' opiate addiction with a replacement therapy
- Women often (falsely) believe they have to be opiate-free to keep their baby and so may try to reduce replacement therapy without medical supervision
- Women should be told that the most important issue is to engage with maternity and social services and not to reduce replacement therapy without medical supervision
- Reduction of methadone/buprenorphine is very difficult during pregnancy; rapid reduction can lead to more problems such as withdrawal, risk-taking behaviour, and an increase in the use of street drugs
- Some women may require more methadone or Subutex® as pregnancy progresses.

Cannabis use

- Class C drug
- Not thought to be teratogenic but may affect fetal growth
- Most widely used illegal drug in the UK—6.8% of 16–59 year olds used cannabis in 2010–11
- In age groups 16–19, 20–24, and 25–29, the proportion reporting use in the past year was 20%, 15%, and 10.1%, respectively.

Cocaine addiction

- Cocaine is associated with miscarriage, low birthweight, preterm birth, increased perinatal morbidity, and disturbed behaviour in newborn babies
- Overall, 2.1% of 16–59 year olds report use in the past year, but usage ranges from 3 to 4.7% in younger age groups (16–29).

Amphetamine addiction

Colloquially: speed, amphetamine sulfate, phet, billy, whizz, sulph, base, paste, dexamphetamine, dexies, Dexedrine®.

- Swallowed, smoked, snorted, or injected
- Associated with growth restriction, preterm delivery, heart defects, central nervous system (CNS) defects, talipes (especially with ectasy), cleft lip and palate
- Overall, 1% of 16–59 year olds report use in the past year but relatively higher in younger age groups (<29).

Ecstasy (MDMA, 3,4-methylenedioxymethamphetamine)

- Limited data on effects on fetus
- Possible increased risk of congenital abnormalities
- Theoretical risks from vasoconstrictive effects
- 3.8% of 16–24 year olds report taking ectasy in the previous year in 2010–11.

General principles about treatment of substance misuse

See Care pathway.

Further reading

Home Office Statistical Bulletin (2011). Drug misuse declared: findings from the 2010/11 British Crime Survey, England and Wales. Available at: <https://www.gov.uk/government/uploads/system/uploads/attachment_data/file/116333/hosb1211.pdf>.

National Institute for Health and Clinical Excellence *(2010). Pregnancy and complex social factors: a model for service provision for pregnant women with complex social factors. NICE clinical guidance 110.* Available at: <http://www.nice.org.uk/nicemedia/live/13167/50822/50822.pdf>.

UK Teratology Information Service (uktis). Range of leaflets can be downloaded from:

<http://www.uktis.org/docs/ALCOHOL.PDF>

<http://www.uktis.org/docs/buprenorphine.pdf>

<http://www.uktis.org/docs/CANNABIS.PDF>

<http://www.uktis.org/docs/COCAINE.PDF>

<http://www.uktis.org/docs/ECSTASY.PDF>

<http://www.uktis.org/docs/HEROIN.PDF>.

Care pathway for substance misuse in pregnancy

At first contact with maternity services, enquire about use of alcohol and recreational drugs, and, if identified, offer referral to substance misuse programme

Multi-agency integrated care delivery

Involving the multidisciplinary team of obstetrician, midwife, paediatric liaison team, drug/alcohol services, social worker or probation officer, GP and health visitor, mental health services, dietician

An integrated care plan should be developed covering the topics:

- Attendance for antenatal care
- Attendance at other specialist services
- Maternal health, including mental health
- Fetal development and well-being—scan for growth restriction
- Current smoking/alcohol/drug/use
- Involvement and support of partner
- Stability of lifestyle/social circumstances/domestic violence/homelessness
- Current or potential risk
- Preparation for labour and delivery
- Preparation for post-natal period and for parenthood
- Future needs to be addressed
- Child protection issues.

Post-natal care

- Continue multidisciplinary support, if necessary
- Implement post-natal plan
- Monitor drug/alcohol use
- Ensure appropriate contraception after birth— consider long-acting reversible contraception.

Multiple pregnancy

Key learning points

Diagnosis—early diagnosis is essential

Screening for Down's syndrome requires specialist attention

Antenatal care should be delivered in a consultant-led environment with access to fetal medicine services

Delivery may be complicated, and senior medical input should be immediately available.

Introduction

Twin pregnancies can result from the fertilization of one egg, which subsequently divides (monozygotic), or from the fertilization of two different eggs (dizygotic). Rates of monozygotic twins are fairly constant throughout the world at 3.5/1000 births, whilst the rate of dizygotic twins varies, depending on race, age, and use of assisted reproductive techniques. In the UK, the rate of dizygotic twins is about twice that of monozygotic twins. Higher-order multiples are much less common: in the UK, there are less than 200 triplet pregnancies each year and less than 20 higher-order multiples.

Diagnosis

Diagnosis is essentially by ultrasound scan (USS). Some patients will have had an early scan because of assisted reproduction or hyperemesis (which can be a symptom of multiple pregnancy), but most will find out for the first time at their dating scan (11–14 weeks). It is important at this stage to be certain about the number of fetuses and also to establish chorionicity (see Figure 1). In dichorionic twins, the membrane between the twins is thicker, especially towards the uterine wall, and is, therefore, described as the lambda (λ) sign. Monochorionic twins have a thinner membrane between them which joins the uterine wall more abruptly and is, therefore, described as the T sign.

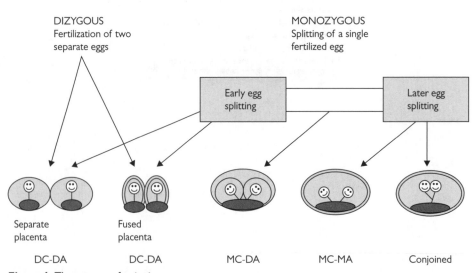

Figure 1 The process of twinning.

Reproduced from Archives of Disease in Childhood Education & Practice, ND Embleton and KVS Pillalamarri, 'Whistle blowing in clinical diagnosis', 92, 3, ep 70–75, Copyright © 2007, with permission from BMJ Publishing Group Ltd and the Royal College of Paediatrics and Child Health.

Screening for Down's syndrome

Screening for Down's syndrome is available in twin pregnancies, using the combined test. However, before embarking on the screening test, patients with dichorionic twins (and, therefore, likely to be dizygous) should consider what they would do if one twin were affected by Down's syndrome and the other were not. Options would include continuing the pregnancy, termination of one twin (with risks to the other), or ending the whole pregnancy.

Antenatal care

Twins and higher-order multiples carry an increased risk of most complications of pregnancy, including:

- Pre-eclampsia
- IUGR
- Preterm labour
- Diabetes
- Post-partum haemorrhage (PPH).

Patients with twins are seen in antenatal clinic up to the end of the second trimester at 4-weekly intervals and subsequently 2-weekly, or more frequently, with urinalysis, blood pressure (BP) measurement, and ultrasound assessment.

Monochorionic twins share the same placenta and, therefore, the same circulation. About 10% of monochorionic twins develop twin-twin transfusion syndrome (TTTS). One fetus becomes hypervolaemic (i.e. transfused), and the other becomes hypovolaemic. In mild cases, this is diagnosed by a discrepancy in liquor volume, as the hypervolaemic fetus increases its urine output and the hypovolaemic fetus decreases its urine output to try and compensate. More severe cases can lead to heart failure or even demise of the fetuses. Not all cases progress to term. Treatment, using fetoscopic laser ablation of the communicating vessels on the placental surface, is available in specialized units, but this is reserved for more severe cases because of the procedure-related risks of miscarriage/preterm labour, membrane rupture, and fetal demise. Monochorionic twins are usually seen every 2 weeks from 16 weeks because of the risk of TTTS.

There are currently no preventative measures in multiple pregnancies to reduce the risk of preterm labour, but patients should be aware that 50% of twins will have been born by 37 weeks, either because of preterm labour or because of complications of pregnancy that have necessitated early delivery.

Delivery

In the absence of indications to deliver earlier, monochorionic twins are usually delivered at 36–37 weeks and dichorionic twins at 37–38 weeks. The main factor to consider when planning mode of delivery is the presentation of the first twin. If non-cephalic, C/S is recommended. Some obstetricians advocate C/S for all twins, or for all monochorionic twins, but there is no robust evidence to support this or indeed the timing of delivery in twins.

Further reading

National Institute for Health and Clinical Excellence (2011). *Multiple pregnancy. The management of twin and triplet pregnancies in the antenatal period.* NICE clinical guideline 129. Available at: <http://www.nice.org.uk/nicemedia/live/13571/56422/56422.pdf>.

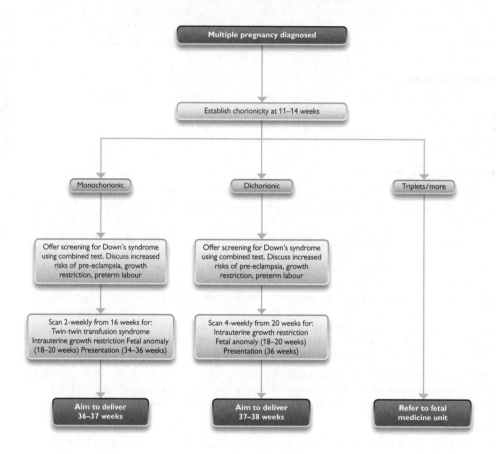

Algorithm for multiple pregnancy

Multiple pregnancy diagnosed

Establish chorionicity at 11–14 weeks

Monochorionic

Offer screening for Down's syndrome using combined test. Discuss increased risks of pre-eclampsia, growth restriction, preterm labour

Scan 2-weekly from 16 weeks for:
Twin-twin transfusion syndrome
Intrauterine growth restriction Fetal anomaly (18–20 weeks) Presentation (34–36 weeks)

Aim to deliver 36–37 weeks

Dichorionic

Offer screening for Down's syndrome using combined test. Discuss increased risks of pre-eclampsia, growth restriction, preterm labour

Scan 4-weekly from 20 weeks for:
Intrauterine growth restriction
Fetal anomaly (18–20 weeks)
Presentation (36 weeks)

Aim to deliver 37–38 weeks

Triplets/more

Refer to fetal medicine unit

Vaginal discharge in pregnancy

Key learning points

Discharge in pregnancy may be physiological or infective

Sexually transmitted disease (STD) must be excluded

Consider membrane rupture.

Definition

- Secretions from the vagina
- Can be physiological or pathological
- Quantity increases in pregnancy
- Can cause concern for the pregnant woman.

Common causes

- Physiological
  - In pregnancy, the vaginal muscle hypertrophies and there is a change in the surrounding connective tissue
  - There is increased shedding of the vaginal mucosal cells
  - These changes are mediated by oestrogen and lead to increased vaginal discharge
  - This discharge is called **leucorrhoea** and is a non-offensive, clear/white, non-infective discharge
- Pathological.

Infective

- Candidiasis (thrush)
  - Fungal infection causing thick, white discharge and vaginal itch. Treated with an imidazole cream or pessary
  - Diagnosed with vaginal swab
  - 5–15% women suffer recurrent infections (≥4 episodes/year)
  - In such cases, consider underlying conditions, e.g. diabetes, immunosuppression
- Bacterial vaginosis
  - Affects 10–20% of women
  - Increased incidence in pregnancy
  - 50% can be asymptomatic
  - Decreased hydrogen peroxide production by lactobacilli in vagina leads to increased vaginal pH
  - Overgrowth of *Gardnerella vaginalis*
  - Thin, grey discharge with 'fishy' odour
  - Microscopy of vaginal swab shows clue cells
  - Treat with metronidazole or clindamycin
  - Can be associated with preterm birth or premature rupture of membranes
  - Screen high-risk women at booking visit
- Chlamydia
  - STI with *Chlamydia trachomatis*
  - Often asymptomatic but can cause mucopurulent discharge
  - Diagnosed using PCR from endocervical swab or first-pass urine
  - Higher incidence in women under age 25
  - Offer screening to all pregnant women
  - Treat with 1 g azithromycin stat dose or 7–14-day course of erythromycin
  - Doxycycline not recommended in pregnancy
  - Treat sexual partners
  - Recommend test of cure

- Gonorrhoea
  - STI with *Neisseria gonorrhoeae*
  - Can be asymptomatic or cause purulent discharge
  - Offer screening to all pregnant women
  - Diagnosed with endocervical swab associated with presence of Gram-negative intracellular diplococci on culture
  - For treatment, check local sensitivities
  - As ciprofloxacin not recommended in pregnancy, often use 250 mg ceftriaxone IM
  - Treat sexual partners
  - Recommend test of cure
- Trichomoniasis
  - Parasitic infection with *Trichomonas vaginalis*
  - Profuse vaginal discharge ± irritation and itchiness of vagina and vulva
  - Associated with preterm labour
  - Diagnosed with vaginal swab
  - Treat with metronidazole 2 g stat dose or 400 mg bd for 7 days
  - Treat sexual partners, and refer to genitourinary medicine (GUM) clinic
  - Recommend test of cure.

Pregnancy-related
- Rupture of the membranes
  - Loss of amniotic fluid
  - Described as a sudden 'gush' of fluid
  - Can be clear, bloodstained, or meconium-stained
  - Management depends on gestation at which it occurs and other obstetric factors
- Show
  - Loss of mucous plug
  - Can be thick mucous, bloodstained discharge
  - Can be associated with start of labour.

Neoplasia
- Rarely, malignancies of the genital tract can complicate pregnancy and lead to vaginal discharge.

Clinical management

Full history, focussing on current symptoms, gestation, risk factors for STDs, and features of the discharge.

Examination

Observations, temperature, abdominal palpation, sterile speculum examination. Assess for abdominal/uterine tenderness, presence of discharge or amniotic fluid. Perform triple swabs for full STD screen, if warranted.

Ongoing management depends on clinical findings.

If features of leucorrhoea, simply reassure the patient.

If features of a show or rupture of the membranes, management depends on gestational age—see relevant chapter.

If features of an STD, treat with the appropriate antibiotics as an outpatient unless clinically unwell. Ensure the patient is aware of risks of preterm labour, and stress upon the importance of completing the course of treatment and for partner(s) to be treated. Alert paediatricians as the baby may need review ± treatment.

If concerns of malignancy, may need imaging, examination under anaesthesia (EUA), or biopsies. Management may depend on gestation. Consider early delivery to aid ongoing investigation ± treatment.

Further reading

Mitchell H (2004). ABC of sexually transmitted infections. Vaginal discharge—causes, diagnosis, and treatment. *BMJ*, **328**, 1306–8.

Care pathway for vaginal discharge in pregnancy

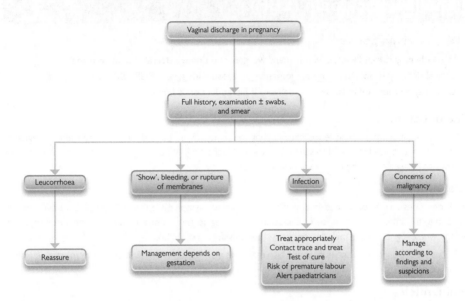

Vaginal discharge in pregnancy

Full history, examination ± swabs, and smear

Leucorrhoea

'Show', bleeding, or rupture of membranes

Infection

Concerns of malignancy

Reassure

Management depends on gestation

Treat appropriately
Contact trace and treat
Test of cure
Risk of premature labour
Alert paediatricians

Manage according to findings and suspicions

Pregnancy-related pelvic girdle pain (PGP) and low back pain (LBP)

Key learning points

Physiotherapy is rapidly effective for many women, and timely referral should be made

Vaginal delivery is possible in most women, even those with severe PGP/LBP

Care may be required in labour and delivery if hip abduction is limited.

Introduction

Many pregnant women experience pain in their pelvis or lower back during, or soon after, pregnancy. Symptoms may range from mild to severe and can be debilitating. Although symptoms are common, it is not normal to have pain that limits a woman's activities of daily living.

Definitions

PGP describes pain experienced in any of the pelvic joints (symphysis pubis and sacroiliac joints), and may extend to the inner thigh, groin, lower back, buttock, hip region, perineum, anterior thigh, or posterior aspect of the whole leg. This term includes 'symphysis pubis dysfunction' (SPD).

LBP describes pain in the lumbar region, which may have a dermatomal distribution. There may be neurological involvement.

Epidemiology

PGP and/or LBP occur in 45–72% of pregnant women. Approximately 25% of pregnant women and 5% of post-partum women require intervention. Untreated, PGP may continue for >2 years. The onset of PGP and/or LBP is often in the second or third trimester. However, symptoms may present at any stage, including immediately following delivery.

Aetiology

The causes of PGP and LBP vary between individuals. Pain is related to biomechanical alterations in the lumbopelvic region, including changes in joint motion and muscle activation patterns. A few women are thought to have hormonally induced pain; they may present earlier in pregnancy with severe pain.

Risk factors

- Previous PGP and/or LBP, including trauma
- High stress, low job satisfaction, strenuous work
- Multiparity
- High body mass index (BMI)
- General joint hypermobility.

Clinical management

Differential diagnosis

- Urinary tract or other infection
- Braxton–Hicks or labour contractions
- Deep vein thrombosis (DVT)
- Inguinal or femoral hernia.

Conditions to be aware of

- Transient osteoporosis of the hip
- Disc prolapse with cauda equina signs
- Diastasis symphysis pubis (DSP)—requires radiological diagnosis after delivery, for women with ongoing PGP. The size of diastasis does not correlate to pain severity.

Referral for treatment

Prompt referral to an experienced obstetric physiotherapist is essential and often resolves symptoms quickly. Women can be treated at any stage of pregnancy or the post-natal period, and those with a history of PGP/LBP should be referred early. Women with severe PGP/LBP may require ongoing input. Treatment modalities include manual therapy, exercise, advice on activities of daily living, provision of maternity belts and walking aids, hydrotherapy, acupuncture, and TENS.

Women may also benefit from osteopathy, chiropractic, and complementary therapies.

Advice and management

- Acknowledge the physical and emotional impact of PGP and/or LBP on the woman and her family
- Ensure appropriate analgesia
- Advise to:
  - Remain active as pain permits—rest for short periods through the day
  - Accept offers of help and support
  - Avoid asymmetrical positions and activities.

Labour and delivery

- Women with severe pain may require counselling about mode of delivery. Most women should be able to have a vaginal delivery. In very severe cases, elective C/S may be considered
- Women with a restriction of bilateral hip abduction: the pain-free range should be recorded in the obstetric notes. Measure the distance between the medial edges of the patellae, with the woman in crook lying and feet together
- Care should be taken to avoid moving beyond the woman's pain-free range of hip abduction (especially with epidural use), unless there is an obstetric indication
- Move legs symmetrically
- Where possible, vaginal examinations and suturing should be performed in the most comfortable position for the woman, e.g. side lying
- Where an instrumental delivery is required, ventouse is preferred; it may be possible to deliver in left lateral position. Unless delivery is likely to be easy, an emergency C/S may be a better option.

Post-partum

- Breastfeeding should be encouraged and is not related to post-partum PGP and/or LBP
- Prescribe appropriate analgesia
- Women who have had severe PGP and/or LBP during pregnancy may be wise to ensure recovery from this pregnancy before planning another baby.

Further reading

Association of Chartered Physiotherapists in Women's Health (ACPWH) (2011). *Pregnancy-related pelvic girdle pain—for health professionals*. Ralph Allen Press, Bath.

Gutke A, Ostgaard HC, Oberg B (2006). Pelvic girdle pain and lumbar pain in pregnancy: a cohort study of the consequences in terms of health and functioning. *Spine*, **31**, E149–55.

Wu WH, Meijer OG, Uegaki K, *et al.* (2004). Pregnancy-related pelvic girdle pain (PPP), I: Terminology, clinical presentation, and prevalence. *European Spine Journal*, **13**, 575–89.

Care pathway for pregnancy-related pelvic girdle pain and low back pain

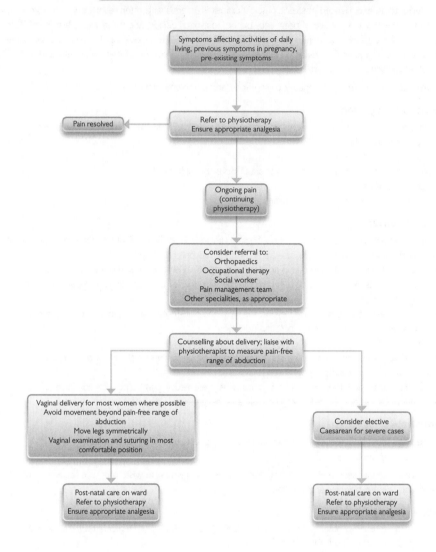

Exercise in pregnancy

Key learning points

When to exercise in pregnancy

Benefits of exercise in pregnancy

Medical supervision of exercise

Prescribing an exercise programme.

Introduction

Exercise during pregnancy helps to manage many minor problems of pregnancy and helps to establish good habits for the woman and her family. Advice on when and how to exercise should be tailored to the individual, based on her general health, obstetric well-being, and exercise history.

Benefits of exercise

In addition to the usual benefits of exercise during pregnancy, exercise may:

- Reduce the incidence of gestational diabetes mellitus
- Aid management of gestational weight gain
- Reduce the rate of C/S
- Help the fetus to tolerate labour better.

Conditions requiring medical supervision include:

- Cardiac/respiratory/orthopaedic conditions
- Poorly controlled hypertension, diabetes mellitus, seizures, thyroid disease, anaemia
- Persistent bleeding, pre-eclampsia, multiple gestation, placenta praevia, cervical weakness, IUGR, current or previous preterm labour, premature ruptured membranes.

Women should stop exercising and seek medical advice if they experience:

- Excessive shortness of breath, chest pain, palpitations, presyncope, dizziness, fatigue
- Abdominal, LBP or PGP, headache, calf pain or swelling
- Painful uterine contractions, preterm labour, reduced fetal movements
- Leakage of amniotic fluid or vaginal bleeding.

Prescribing an exercise programme—general advice

- Exercise intensity should be 'somewhat hard'. Women should be able to hold a conversation whilst exercising
- Include warm-up and cool-down
- Appropriate forms of exercise include swimming, walking, cycling, pregnancy-specific exercise classes
- Avoid hyperthermia—ensure adequate fluid and calorie intake; avoid exercising in hot humid conditions
- Practise regular pelvic floor muscle exercises.

Sedentary (non-regular exercisers)

- Maximal training heart rate of 60–70% of maximum
- Initially, 15 min of continuous exercise three times per week, progressing as able.

Regular and elite exercisers

- Maximal training heart rate of 60–90% of maximum
- Modification of existing training regime
- Expect a gradual decline in fitness levels and ability as pregnancy advances
- Regular monitoring if elite, and advice on hydration, nutrition, dangers of heat stress.

Post-natal

- Uncomplicated vaginal delivery—start low-impact exercise as soon as woman feels able
- C/S or complicated vaginal delivery—walk within comfort; wait until post-natal check up (6–8 weeks) before doing further exercise
- Practise regular pelvic floor muscle exercises.

Further reading

Artal R, O'Toole M, White S (2003). Guidelines of the American College of Obstetricians and Gynecologists for exercise during pregnancy and the postpartum period. *British Journal of Sports Medicine*, **37**, 6–12.

National Institute for Health and Clinical Excellence (2008). *Antenatal care: routine care for the healthy pregnant women.* NICE clinical guideline 62. Available at: <http://www.nice.org.uk/nicemedia/pdf/cg062niceguideline.pdf>.

Royal College of Obstetricians and Gynaecologists (2006). *Exercise in pregnancy.* RCOG Press, London.

Streuling I, Beyerlein A, Rosenfeld E, Hofmann H, Schulz T, von Kries R (2011). Physical activity and gestational weight gain: a meta-analysis of intervention trials. *British Journal of Obstetrics and Gynaecology*, **118**, 278–84.

Care pathway for exercise in pregnancy

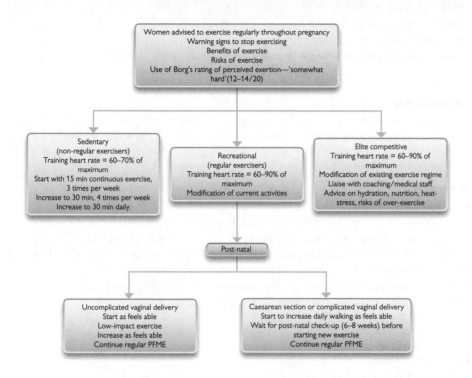

Women advised to exercise regularly throughout pregnancy
Warning signs to stop exercising
Benefits of exercise
Risks of exercise
Use of Borg's rating of perceived exertion—'somewhat hard'(12–14/20)

Sedentary
(non-regular exercisers)
Training heart rate = 60–70% of maximum
Start with 15 min continuous exercise, 3 times per week
Increase to 30 min, 4 times per week
Increase to 30 min daily

Recreational
(regular exercisers)
Training heart rate = 60–90% of maximum
Modification of current activities

Elite competitive
Training heart rate = 60–90% of maximum
Modification of existing exercise regime
Liaise with coaching/medical staff
Advice on hydration, nutrition, heat-stress, risks of over-exercise

Post-natal

Uncomplicated vaginal delivery
Start as feels able
Low-impact exercise
Increase as feels able
Continue regular PFME

Caesarean section or complicated vaginal delivery
Start to increase daily walking as feels able
Wait for post-natal check-up (6–8 weeks) before starting new exercise
Continue regular PFME

Travelling in pregnancy

Key learning points

When to travel in pregnancy

Risks with travelling in pregnancy

How to minimize risks associated with travelling in pregnancy.

Introduction

Most women with a healthy pregnancy can travel safely. According to the American College of Obstetrics and Gynecology, the best time to travel is between 14 and 28 weeks of pregnancy. In the first 12 weeks of pregnancy, there is a higher risk of miscarriage or ectopic pregnancy. After 28 weeks, the biggest issue with travel is the risk of preterm labour.

Air travel

- Consider quality of medical care at the destination
- Arrange appropriate medical insurance, vaccination, and malaria prophylaxis.

The discrepancy between the aircraft environment and the ground environment relates to the atmosphere. Modern aircraft are not pressurized to a sea level equivalent. The cabin altitude will be between 1524 m and 2438 m. Thus, the barometric pressure is significantly lower than at sea level.

- Reduced barometric pressure in aircraft cabin causes a reduction in blood oxygen saturation by 10% which is compensated by favourable properties of fetal haemoglobin (Hb):
  - Increased oxygen carrying affinity
  - Increased fetal haematocrit
  - The Bohr effect
- Low cabin humidity (10–20%)
  - Drying effect on airways, the cornea, and the skin
- Risk of deep venous thrombosis (DVT)
  - Aircraft seating is cramped, and passengers tend to remain immobile
  - Risk increased by presence of additional risk factors such as previous DVT or obesity
  - Risk decreased by regular walks every hour or two
  - Risk decreased with graduated elastic compression stocking.

A recent World Health Organization (WHO) study in non-pregnant individuals described a 2–4-fold increased risk of new thrombosis associated with air travel. A Cochrane review reported that graduated elastic compression stocking would significantly reduce the risk of asymptomatic DVT. RCOG recommends that, if the woman has additional risk factors for thrombosis, such as a previous DVT, morbid obesity, or medical problems, such as nephrotic syndrome, specific pharmacological prophylaxis with low-molecular-weight heparin (LMWH) in the doses recommended for antenatal prophylaxis should be considered for the day of travel and several days thereafter.

- Risk of delivery in the aircraft
  - Many airlines do not allow women to fly after 36 completed weeks of gestation
  - Women with multiple pregnancies should not fly after 33 completed weeks of gestation
- Risk of radiation
  - Earth's atmosphere absorbs much of the cosmic radiation
  - At the airliner altitudes, there is much less atmosphere, therefore, radiation levels are greater than at the sea level.

The US department of transportation stated that commercial pilots and aircrew exposure to cosmic radiation do not indicate excessive radiation doses, compared to occupational radiation limits in industry. According to Aerospace Medical Association, expectant mothers should not be considered to be at increased risk, unless they are flying several times a week during their pregnancy.

Further reading

Aerospace Medical Association Medical Guidelines Task Force (2003). Medical Guidelines for Airline Travel, 2nd ed. *Aviation, Space, and Environmental Medicine*, **74** (5 Suppl), A1–19.

American College of Obstetricians and Gynecologists (2011). *Travel during pregnancy.* Available at: <http://www.acog.org/~/media/For%20Patients/faq055.pdf?dmc=1&ts=20131008T1056545290>.

http://www.acog.org/publications/patient_education/bp055.cfm

Royal College of Obstetricians and Gynaecologist (2008). *Air travel and pregnancy.* Scientific Advisory Committee Opinion Paper 1. Available at: <http://www.rcog.org.uk/files/rcog-corp/uploaded-files/SAC1AirTravelPregnancy2008.pdf>.

US Department of Transportation, Federal Aviation Administration (1990). *Radiation exposure of air carrier crewmembers.* Advisory circular. Available at: <http://www.airweb.faa.gov/Regulatory_and_Guidance_Library/rgAdvisoryCircular.nsf/0/4429e431e6426faf862569bc0057cd44/$FILE/ATTTZXZ6/AC120-52.pdf>.

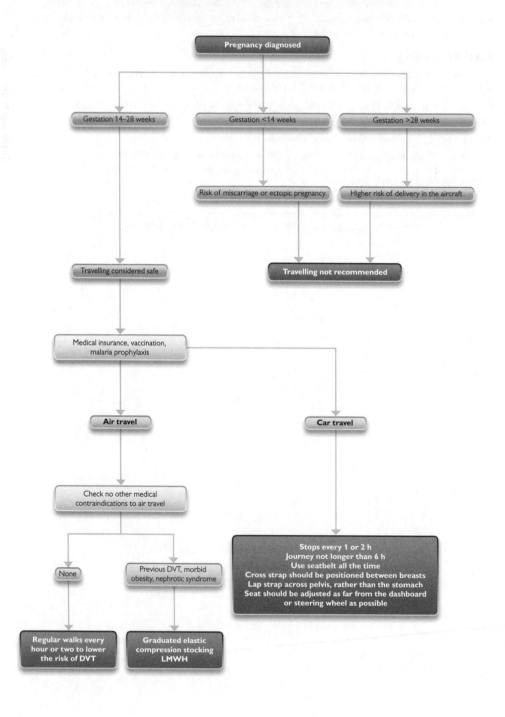

Algorithm for travelling in pregnancy

Pregnancy diagnosed

Gestation 14–28 weeks

Gestation <14 weeks

Gestation >28 weeks

Risk of miscarriage or ectopic pregnancy

Higher risk of delivery in the aircraft

Travelling considered safe

Travelling not recommended

Medical insurance, vaccination, malaria prophylaxis

Air travel

Car travel

Check no other medical contraindications to air travel

None

Previous DVT, morbid obesity, nephrotic syndrome

Stops every 1 or 2 h
Journey not longer than 6 h
Use seatbelt all the time
Cross strap should be positioned between breasts
Lap strap across pelvis, rather than the stomach
Seat should be adjusted as far from the dashboard
or steering wheel as possible

Regular walks every hour or two to lower the risk of DVT

Graduated elastic compression stocking LMWH

Management of constipation

Key learning points

Constipation is a common symptom of pregnancy

Evaluation should attempt to distinguish between slow transit and obstructive constipation

Treatment should initially address diet and may include laxative agents.

Introduction

Constipation is a symptom of many conditions. The commonest definitions are infrequent passage of stools (<2/week), straining >25% of time, passage of hard stools, and incomplete evacuation. It is estimated to affect >20% of the population.

Causes

- Functional
  - Pregnancy, low-fibre intake, immobility, irritable bowel syndrome (IBS), and idiopathic slow transit
- Psychological
  - Repressed urge to defecate—chronic pain, anorexia nervosa, and depression
- Gastrointestinal (GI) disease
  - Intestinal obstruction, solitary ulcer syndrome, pseudo-obstruction, anal fissure, colonic carcinoma, and megarectum
- Metabolic/endocrine diseases
  - Hypothyroidism, hypercalcaemia, diabetes mellitus, and porphyria
- Neurological disorders
  - Spinal cord lesions and Parkinson's disease
- Drugs
  - Opiates, anticholinergics, calcium channel blockers, antidepressants, and iron
- Obstructive disorders
  - Rectal prolapse, intussusception, Hirschprung's disease, large rectocele, and pelvic floor dysfunction.

Evaluation

Most causes of constipation can be identified by a careful history. A recent change in bowel habit, in association with other symptoms, such as rectal bleeding, requires urgent investigation. This will usually involve a barium enema, sigmoidoscopy, or colonoscopy. A barium enema should always be preceded by a rectal examination and rigid sigmoidoscopy to exclude anorectal lesions.

The two clinical types of constipation are slow transit and obstructive. In the slow-transit form, patients rarely experience a call to stool. In the obstructive form, patients experience a call to stool but are not able to evacuate properly because of coexisting organic and functional anorectal disease.

A simple abdominal X-ray and marker studies of colonic transit can assess the severity of slow-transit constipation. Obstructive constipation is assessed by performing evacuation proctography.

Treatment

Laxatives, in combination with increasing fibre, fluid intake, and physical activity levels, are usually effective and should be tailored to the needs of the patient. Macrogols are suitable for titration according to clinical effect.

Regular treatment is more effective than ad hoc use, and stimulant laxatives should be used cautiously. Excessive use of laxatives may lead to electrolyte disturbances.

Types of laxatives

- Bulk-forming laxatives—relieve constipation by increasing faecal mass which stimulates peristalsis. The full effect may take some days to develop. They include methylcellulose, ispaghula, and sterculia

- Osmotic laxatives—act by increasing colonic inflow of fluid and electrolyte which soften stool and stimulate colonic contractility. They include lactulose, macrogols, magnesium salts, and phosphate enemas
- Stimulant laxatives—increase intestinal motility and often cause abdominal cramp; they should be avoided in intestinal obstruction. Excessive use can cause diarrhoea and related effects such as hypokalaemia. They include bisacodyl, dantron, docusate sodium, glycerol, senna, and sodium picosulfate
- Faecal softeners—these preparations contain oil which soften stool. These include arachis oil and liquid paraffin.

Further reading

Lindsay J, Langmead L, Preston SL (2012). Gastrointestinal disease. In P Kumar and M Clark, eds. *Clinical Medicine*, pp. 229–302, 8th edn. Saunders Elsevier, UK.

National Institute for Health and Clinical Excellence (2010). *Constipation in children and young people*. NICE clinical guideline 99. Available at: <http://www.nice.org.uk/nicemedia/live/12993/48741/48741.pdf>.

Care pathway for the management of constipation

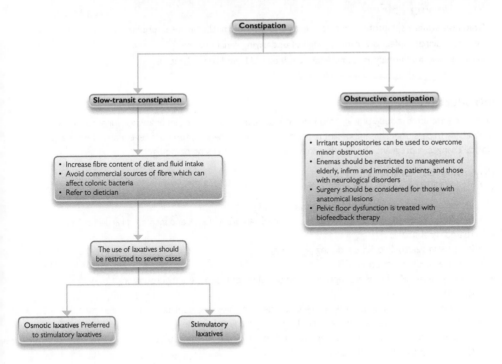

Constipation

Slow-transit constipation

- Increase fibre content of diet and fluid intake
- Avoid commercial sources of fibre which can affect colonic bacteria
- Refer to dietician

The use of laxatives should be restricted to severe cases

Osmotic laxatives Preferred to stimulatory laxatives

Stimulatory laxatives

Obstructive constipation

- Irritant suppositories can be used to overcome minor obstruction
- Enemas should be restricted to management of elderly, infirm and immobile patients, and those with neurological disorders
- Surgery should be considered for those with anatomical lesions
- Pelvic floor dysfunction is treated with biofeedback therapy

Urinary tract symptoms in pregnancy

Key learning points

Common urinary symptoms are often related to physiological changes in pregnancy

Repeated urinary infections can be a sign of underlying renal disease

Routine antenatal urinalysis is important to detect UTI and pre-eclampsia.

Introduction

Common symptoms include urinary frequency, nocturia, dysuria, urgency, incontinence (urgency and stress), and inability to pass urine. It is important to identify whether these symptoms are reflections of normal physiological changes in pregnancy or whether they represent an underlying pathology.

Physiological changes

- Small increase in urine output
  - Increase in renal perfusion and glomerular filtration rate
  - Resulting from widespread vasodilation, increased vascular volume, and increased cardiac output
- Increased renal size
  - Increase in size by 1 to 1.5 cm during pregnancy
  - Increase in volume of up to 30%
- Dilation of renal pelvices (hydronephrosis) and dilatation of the ureters (hydroureter)
  - Causes:
    o High progesterone levels reduce ureteric tone, peristalsis, and contraction pressure
    o Mechanical compression at the pelvic brim—right side > left side
    o Uterine enlargement causes elongation and lateral displacement of ureters
  - Occurs in up to 80% of pregnancies
  - Commonly asymptomatic
  - Right side is affected more than the left
  - Results in increased volume of urine in the collecting system (200–300 mL)
    o Reservoir of urine
    o Increased risk of pyelonephritis and UTI
- Bladder changes
  - Progesterone-induced bladder wall relaxation can increase capacity
  - Compression from enlarging uterus causes displacement and reduced capacity
- Intermittent vesicoureteric reflux
  - Causes:
    o Incompetence of the vesicoureteral valve
    o Increased intravesical pressure
    o Decreased intraureteral pressure
- Biochemical changes—fall in serum creatinine and urea due to increased renal plasma flow.

History and symptoms

See Key information.

- Frequency
  - Definition: voiding >7 times a day
  - Very common
  - Typically begins in first trimester
  - Causes are multifactorial:
    o Mechanical factors mentioned previously
    o Increased urine output

- Nocturia
  - Definition: voiding ≥2 times a night
  - Increases with advanced gestation
  - Causes:
    - Greater excretion of sodium and water at night, compared with non-pregnant women
    - Mobilization of dependent oedema when lying down
- Dysuria
  - Painful urination
  - During and/or after urination
- Urgency and incontinence
  - Urgency—a sudden desire to pass urine which is difficult to defer
  - Urge incontinence—a sudden urge to urinate, followed by incontinence
  - Stress incontinence—an episode of incontinence with activities resulting in increases in intra-abdominal pressure, e.g. cough, laugh, exercising. Due to:
    - Current pregnancy (temporary)
    - Previous childbirth and pelvic floor damage (potentially resulting in permanent problems)
- Inability to pass urine (retention)
  - Frequent small volumes of urine, suggestive of incomplete emptying
  - Followed by an acute episode of retention
  - Causes:
    - Approximately 16 weeks' gestation with incarceration of the retroverted uterus (pressure on the bladder neck with elongation of the urethra)
    - In labour due to deeply engaged head
    - With UTI
- Bloodstained urine (haematuria)
  - Presence of red blood cells in the urine
  - Often difficult to distinguish from liquor if it occurs with membrane rupture
  - Microscopic or macroscopic
- Foul-smelling, concentrated urine
  - Common presentation for UTI.

Physical examination

- Routine observations—to identify pyrexia or signs of sepsis
- Abdominal findings: pain either suprapubic, bilateral, or unilateral flank
- Urine inspection.

Investigations

- Urine tests: urinalysis
  - Urine test strip—to assess for leucocytes, nitrite, protein, blood, ketone bodies, glucose, bilirubin, specific gravity, and pH
  - Midstream urine sample (MSU)
    - Microscopy—to assess for haematuria, pyuria, red or white cell casts
    - Microbiological culture
- Renal tract USS
- Catheterization—to test for retention
- Urine output charts
- Biochemistry—blood serum electrolytes, urea and creatinine assessment to assess renal function.

Differential diagnoses

- UTI
  - Acute cystitis—treat with 5 days' antibiotics (ensure urine MSU is requested)
  - Acute pyelonephritis—for IV antibiotics if pyrexic or no response to oral antibiotics

- Recurrent infection—prophylactic low-dose once-daily antibiotics. Can represent an underlying renal tract pathology
- Ureteric or renal calculi (stones)—leading to renal colic (presentation is as in non-pregnant population)
- Hydronephrosis or hydroureters
  - Due to physiological changes or calculi
  - For urological team review if symptomatic
- Urinary retention—due to:
  - Mechanical changes or obstruction: retroverted uterus in first trimester, compression from presenting part in labour
  - Infection
- ASB (asymptomatic bacteriuria)
  - 5% of pregnant women have asymptomatic, previously unidentified urinary infection
  - 30% of which will go on to develop symptomatic infections
    - Increased risk of pregnancy complications (premature labour, IUGR, pre-eclampsia).
  - Important for regular antenatal urinalysis screening.

Further reading

Vazquez JC and Abalos E (2011). Treatments for symptomatic urinary tract infections during pregnancy. *Cochrane Database of Systematic Reviews*, **1**, CD002256.

Key information for the interpretation of urinary tract symptoms and signs in pregnancy

Symptom/sign	Physiological	Physiological but requiring treatment	Pathological
Frequency	✔	✘	✔
Nocturia	✔	✘	✔
Dysuria	✘	✘	✔
Urgency	✔	✘	✔
Incontinence	✔	✘	✔
Retention	✔	✔	✔
Incomplete emptying	✔	✔	✔
Haematuria	✘	✘	✔

Rhesus alloimmunization

Key learning points

Mechanism of rhesus (Rh) sensitization

Prophylaxis with routine administration of anti-D

Management of the sensitized fetus.

Introduction

- Rh disease remains a serious obstetric challenge, particularly in countries without an organized antenatal prophylaxis programme
- Less common in the UK since the introduction of immunoprophylaxis in 1969
- No prophylaxis against other (non-Rh) red cell alloimmunity (similar management strategies).

Pathophysiology

All erythrocytes display surface antigens. About 15% of the UK population lack the Rh antigen (Rh-negative). Exposure to 'foreign' fetal erythrocyte antigens via a fetomaternal haemorrhage (FMH) may trigger an immune response (also termed sensitization). This process is called alloimmunization (formerly isoimmunization). This may occur at childbirth, following trauma or an APH but can also occur 'silently' without any obvious clinical features. A repeat antigen exposure (perhaps in a subsequent pregnancy) can provoke a larger maternal anti-body response. The active transport of these maternal antibodies across the placenta can cause fetal anaemia, hyperbilirubinaemia, hydrops fetalis, and death. This process is termed haemolytic disease of the fetus and newborn (HDFN). There are many antigens which can provoke this process, of which the commonest is the Rh antigen (Rh disease is the term often used). Others systems include Kell, Duffy, MNS, Kidd anti-U.

Prophylaxis

- In the UK, Rh prophylaxis was introduced in 1969. Deaths attributed to RhD alloimmunization fell from 46/100 000 to 1.6/100 000 births by 1990
- A dose of 500 IU of anti-D immunoglobulin will bind to fetal Rh antigens and neutralize up to 4 mL of Rh-positive fetal blood, preventing maternal sensitization
- Rh antigen and erthyrocyte antibody status is assessed at booking, and non-sensitized Rh-negative women are offered immunoprophylaxis (women who are already sensitized will not benefit)
- Following negative repeat erythrocyte antibody testing, an IM injection of immunoglobulin (collected from Rh-negative donors) is given at 28 weeks' gestation
- Rh-negative women are also offered additional immunoprophylaxis after potential sensitizing events— anything which could involve FMH, including childbirth (where the baby is Rh-positive), trauma, APH, stillbirth, miscarriage or ectopic pregnancy, manual removal of placenta, and invasive procedures such as amniocentesis and CVS
- Regimens vary from country to country (minimum 250 IU before 20 weeks and 500 IU after 20 weeks)
- 250 IU at 28 weeks in the UK
- Anti-D should be given as soon as possible within 72 h of the event
- After delivery, the baby's Rh status should be established by a cord blood sample. If the baby is Rh-positive (around 60% will be), further anti-D should be given, and a test to determine the degree of FMH should be taken (Kleihauer or modern automated test)
- Additional anti-D may be required, if the result indicates significant FMH, on haematological advice.

Rhesus disease

- No prophylaxis or failure leads to development of Rh antibodies
- Refer to a fetal medicine subspecialist
- Antibody level quantified by a reference lab. Repeated testing as advised by lab

- Fetal Rh status can be predicted with 96.5% accuracy by free fetal DNA analysis. Prediction of an Rh-negative fetus is relatively reassuring
- Predicted Rh-positive fetus, combined with rapid increases in antibody levels, particularly at early gestations, is ominous
- Fetal anaemia can be predicted non-invasively by Doppler ultrasound measurement of fetal blood flow. Hyperdynamic flow in the middle cerebral artery (MCA) occurs in anaemic fetuses
- Fetuses with significant anaemia can benefit from *in utero* blood transfusion (IUT). A needle is passed, under ultrasound direct vision, into either the umbilical vein within the fetal abdomen or in the umbilical cord. A blood sample is taken to determine the haematocrit, and blood is transfused. The volume transfused is determined by gestation and fetal and donor haematocrits
- IUT is a relatively high-risk invasive procedure, with a 5–10% risk of serious complications, including fetal death. IUT may be required weekly in severe cases
- Affected fetuses are generally delivered at 34 weeks, as the risks of IUT then exceed those of prematurity.

Further reading

National Institute for Health and Clinical Excellence (2008). *Routine antenatal anti-D prophylaxis for women who are rhesus D negative.* Review of NICE technology appraisal guidance 41. Available at: <http://www.nice.org.uk/nicemedia/pdf/ta156guidance.pdf>.

Royal College of Obstetricians and Gynaecologists (2011). *The use of anti-D immunoglobulin for rhesus D prophylaxis.* Green-top guideline No. 22. Available at: <http://www.rcog.org.uk/files/rcog-corp/GTG22AntiDJuly2013.pdf>.

Care pathway for rhesus alloimmunization

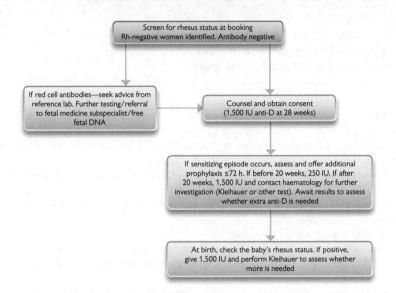

Screen for rhesus status at booking
Rh-negative women identified. Antibody negative

If red cell antibodies—seek advice from reference lab. Further testing/referral to fetal medicine subspecialist/free fetal DNA

Counsel and obtain consent
(1,500 IU anti-D at 28 weeks)

If sensitizing episode occurs, assess and offer additional prophylaxis ≤72 h. If before 20 weeks, 250 IU. If after 20 weeks, 1,500 IU and contact haematology for further investigation (Kleihauer or other test). Await results to assess whether extra anti-D is needed

At birth, check the baby's rhesus status. If positive, give 1,500 IU and perform Kleihauer to assess whether more is needed

Thyroid disease and pregnancy

Key learning points

Thyroid metabolism changes as a result of normal pregnancy

Effects of hypo- and hyperthyroidism in pregnancy

Principles of treating thyroid disorders in pregnancy.

Physiology

- Thyroid-binding globulin is increased in pregnancy; hence a 50% increase in total thyroxine (T4) production is required in order to maintain the functional free T4 concentration in the normal range
- Maternal iodine requirements are increased because of active transport to the fetus and increased maternal renal excretion, with increased uptake of iodine from the maternal blood. If there is dietary insufficiency, this may result in goitre and hypothyroidism
- Thyroid-stimulating hormone (TSH) varies in pregnancy, rising then falling in the first trimester, and then increasing slightly in late pregnancy
- Free T4 is lower in pregnancy
- hCG is structurally similar to TSH, hence the first trimester production of hCG stimulates free T4 production. Conditions with high hCG (molar pregnancy and hyperemesis gravidarum) may, therefore, have transient biochemical hyperthyroidism
- Fetal thyroid hormone synthesis starts at 12 weeks' gestation. Prior to this time, the fetus is dependent on maternal thyroid hormones, becoming gradually less so as pregnancy progresses. Thyroid hormones are important for fetal brain development. The fetus is dependent on maternal iodine throughout pregnancy.

Hyperthyroidism

- Complicates about 0.2% of pregnancies
- Is usually autoimmune in origin, known as Graves's disease
- Is associated with TSH receptor-stimulating antibodies (TRAb). Antibodies can cross the placenta and cause neonatal thyrotoxicosis
- Tends to improve in pregnancy, and many will reduce or stop their antithyroid drugs. Relapse is common post-natally
- Untreated thyrotoxicosis is associated with infertility, miscarriage, IUGR, preterm labour, and perinatal loss. Thyroid storm is a serious maternal complication
- Fetal thyrotoxicosis presents with tachycardia, IUGR, goitre, and perinatal death
- Carbimazole and propylthiouracil (PTU) both cross the placenta and potentially affect the fetal thyroid: doses used should be the lowest required to keep the T4 at the top of the normal range
- Carbimazole has been associated with fetal aplasia cutis; hence PTU is preferred in the first trimester
- Block-and-replace regimes are not appropriate in pregnancy
- Both are excreted in breast milk, but PTU is largely protein-bound and is preferred
- Surgery is occasionally indicated
- Radioactive iodine is contraindicated in pregnancy.

Hypothyroidism

- Is common, complicating about 1% of pregnancies
- Most cases in the UK are autoimmune, but worldwide iodine deficiency is the leading cause
- Inadequate replacement if severe; results in infertility, miscarriage, pre-eclampsia, and stillbirth
- Milder forms of thyroid dysfunction have been associated with neurodevelopmental delay
- Consideration should be given to the cause of hypothyroidsim: women with Graves's disease treated by radioactive iodine or surgery may have TRAbs.

Treatment

- Adequate replacement from early in pregnancy, aiming to keep TSH <2.5 mmol/L
- If adequately replaced, the pregnancy is usually unaffected by hypothyroidism
- Because of the increase in thyroxine synthesis in normal pregnancies, many authorities recommend an increase in thyroxine supplementation from the diagnosis of pregnancy
- Thyroid function, if adequately replaced, should be checked each trimester but, when found to be deficient and increased, checked at 6-weekly intervals
- Thyroxine replacement does not cause fetal thyrotoxicosis
- Fetal hypothyroidism is rare.

Post-partum thyroiditis

- Is due to a rebound in autoimmunity post-delivery
- Presents with transient thyrotoxicosis, followed by transient hypothyroidism, although the former may not be recognized
- Is present in up to 17% of women and classically presents at 3–4 months post-partum
- Diagnosis may be confused with post-natal depression
- Treatment with thyroxine is appropriate but does not need to be lifelong.

Further reading

Nelson-Piercy C (2010). Thyroid and parathyroid disease. In *Handbook of obstetric medicine*, 4th edn, pp. 95–111. Informa Healthcare, London.

Care pathways for thyroid disease and pregnancy

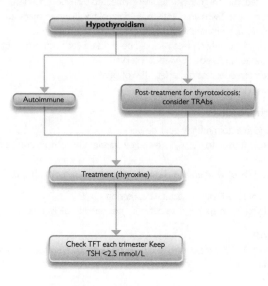

Care pathways for thyroid disease and pregnancy

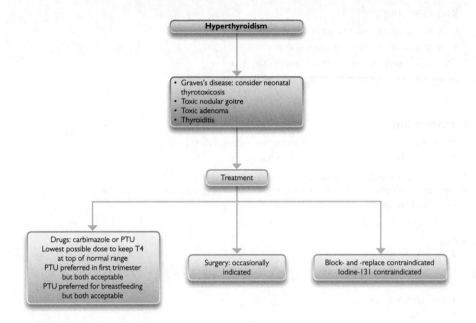

Hyperthyroidism

- Graves's disease: consider neonatal thyrotoxicosis
- Toxic nodular goitre
- Toxic adenoma
- Thyroiditis

Treatment

Drugs: carbimazole or PTU
Lowest possible dose to keep T4 at top of normal range
PTU preferred in first trimester but both acceptable
PTU preferred for breastfeeding but both acceptable

Surgery: occasionally indicated

Block- and -replace contraindicated
Iodine-131 contraindicated

Diabetes mellitus and pregnancy

Key learning points

Diagnosis of gestational diabetes

Effect of pregnancy on established diabetes

Effect of diabetes on the pregnant woman and fetus

Management delivered in a multispecialty environment.

Introduction

Diabetes mellitus is the most common important maternal disease affecting pregnancy, with important consequences to both the mother and child. It includes:

- Pre-existing diabetes mellitus (types 1 and 2)
- Gestational diabetes: disordered glucose metabolism arising during pregnancy, usually a transient abnormality, reverting to normal post-natally.

Adverse outcomes include:

- Fetal
  - Premature delivery
  - Congenital abnormality (most commonly, congenital heart disease and neural tube disorders)
  - Macrosomia
  - Shoulder dystocia
  - Stillbirth
- Maternal
  - Increased risks of pre-eclampsia
  - C/S.

Pathophysiology

Maternal fasting blood glucose is lower than in the non-pregnant state. Post-prandial glucose responses to feeding in late pregnancy are increased and delayed, in comparison to the non-pregnant state, and insulin levels are higher. There is increased insulin sensitivity in early pregnancy and increased insulin resistance in late pregnancy. Glucose is freely transported across the placenta by facilitated diffusion; hence, maternal hyperglycaemia results in fetal hyperinsulinaemia. This acts as an anabolic stimulus, promoting fetal growth. Poor control, therefore, is associated with increased rates of macrosomia and, equally, increased rates of congenital abnormality and stillbirth. The exact mechanism of stillbirth is not known but is associated with chronic fetal hypoxia. Euglycaemia is shown to reduce the rates of abnormality, miscarriage, stillbirth, and macrosomia.

Pattern of care

Preconception care

- Optimize blood glucose control and achieve a euglycaemic state. This will reduce the risk of congenital abnormalies
- Contraception should be discontinued when good control is achieved
- Prescribe folic acid (5 mg).

Antenatal care

- Arrange care in a multidisciplinary environment, with diabetologists, obstetricians, specialist midwives and/or specialist nurses, and dieticians
- Care is intensive, with frequent contact throughout pregnancy
- An early dating scan
- Screen for fetal abnormality, with particular emphasis on neural tube defects (NTDs) and congenital heart disease

- Insulin is the most common hypoglycaemic, although oral hypoglycaemics can be used
- Women are encouraged to test their own blood glucose with home monitors 4–6 times daily, with manipulation of insulin requirements according to changing requirements
- Hypoglycaemia is a particular risk, as awareness of hypoglycaemia may be lost in the first trimester
- Dietary control is essential
- Aspirin administration may help to prevent pre-eclampsia
- Nephropathy and retinopathy, both of which can progress, must be assessed
- Hypertension should be treated and pre-eclampsia promptly diagnosed
- In view of the risk of macrosomia and late intrauterine fetal death (IUFD), fetal surveillance, usually with serial ultrasound, is indicated. There is no proven benefit of a particular regime for assessment of fetal well-being in the third trimester
- Care should be taken to maintain glycaemic control, should administration of antenatal steroids become necessary to promote fetal lung maturity.

Delivery

- NICE guidelines recommend delivery at 38 weeks to prevent late IUFD
- Shoulder dystocia is a particular risk for the infants of diabetic mothers, particularly with fetal macrosomia
- C/S rates are higher in diabetic pregnancies
- Neonatal hypoglycaemia is directly related to maternal blood glucose control in labour; hence, blood glucose must be controlled in labour. This is often with a glucose and insulin infusion for pre-gestational diabetics
- Maternal insulin requirements return promptly to their pre-pregnancy levels immediately post-delivery.

Neonatal implications

- Prematurity rates are high, which, in association with a specific effect of fetal hyperinsulinaemia on the maturation of fetal lungs, results in respiratory distress syndrome
- Fetal hyperinsulinaemia results in neonatal hypoglycaemia which normalizes within a few days of age
- Early infant feeding and blood glucose testing are mandatory
- Polycythaemia, hyperbilirubinaemia, hypocalcaemia, and hypomagnesaemia are also present but, if well controlled, are not usually clinically significant
- Macrosomia can result in birth trauma
- Hypertrophic cardiomyopathy is recognized but uncommon
- The risk of type 1 diabetes in later life is 1.3% if the mother has type 1 diabetes, 6.1% if the father has type 1 diabetes.

Gestational diabetes

Defined as glucose intolerance first diagnosed during pregnancy. Most commonly, it resolves post-pregnancy but identifies women at higher risk of developing type 2 diabetes. However, increasing numbers of those first diagnosed during pregnancy have pre-existing, undiagnosed type 2 or, rarely, type 1 diabetes.

- Diagnosis is usually made with a glucose tolerance test (GTT) at 26–28 weeks
- Aim to achieve euglycaemia, initially with diet, but, if necessary, with metformin and/or insulin
- Principles of care are as for a pre-gestational diabetic; however, the degree of risk is less and related to the time of onset
- Additional risk factors for gestational diabetes mellitus (GDM) include obesity, maternal age, and ethnicity (especially South East Asian)
- A GTT 6 weeks post-natally is indicated to ensure normal glucose handling. In a largely Caucasian population, 20% will remain abnormal.

Further reading

National Institute for Health and Clinical Excellence (2008). *Diabetes in pregnancy: management of diabetes and its complications from pre-conception to the postnatal period.* NICE clinical guideline 63. Available at: <http://www.nice.org.uk/nicemedia/pdf/cg063guidance.pdf>.

Care pathway for diabetes and pregnancy

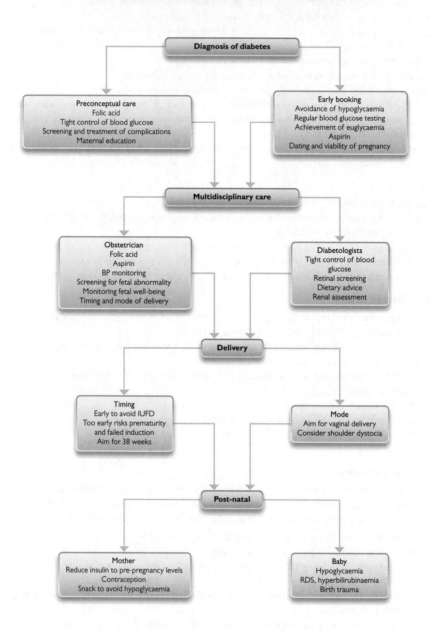

Key learning points

Significant changes in renal physiology occur in pregnancy

Asymptomatic bacteriuria (ASB) may progress to infection

Existing renal disease may lead to increased risks to mother and fetus.

Background

The urinary collecting system is markedly dilated in pregnancy. This is due to the progesterone-mediated smooth muscle relaxation of the ureters and compression by the enlarging uterus. This 'physiological hydronephrosis' is greater on the maternal right side.

The renal plasma flow, glomerular filtration rate, and creatinine clearance all increase early in pregnancy, resulting in lower serum urea and creatinine levels. Physiological sodium and water retention lead to oedema.

Urinary tract infections (UTIs)

ASB is common, affecting 4–7% of pregnant women. Of these, up to 40% will become symptomatic, and some will go on to develop pyelonephritis if untreated. *Escherichia coli* is the most common organism and results from ascending infection from the colonized perineum. The diagnosis is made on a mid-stream urine (MSU) specimen, with a 10^5/mL pure culture of the organism. Dipsticks positive for nitrites and/or leucocytes are suggestive, but not diagnostic, of UTI.

Even ASB should be treated with appropriate antibiotics, e.g. oral cephalosporin or nitrofurantoin, to avoid the risk of pyelonephritis. Repeated proven episodes of infection should result in long-term prophylaxis at night. Women with pyelonephritis are clinically very unwell and may have rigors. There is an association with preterm labour and delivery. Differential diagnoses should be considered, e.g. pulmonary embolism (PE), appendicitis. Ultrasound scanning of the renal tract is merited to exclude congenital or acquired abnormalities, e.g. calculi. IV antibiotic treatment for at least 24 h is indicated. This should be followed by 2 weeks of oral treatment and follow-up urine cultures.

Chronic renal disease

This can be looked at from several viewpoints:

1. The effect of the pregnancy on the chronic renal disease (see Key information)
2. The effect of the degree of renal impairment on the pregnancy outcome (see Key information).

In general, women without hypertension prenatally will do better. There are many different causes of chronic renal disease. The specific underlying maternal pathology also influences the prognosis, e.g. women with diabetic nephropathy do comparatively worse.

Careful preconceptual counselling, preferably by a multidisciplinary team, is vital. Patients need to be stabilized on 'pregnancy-friendly' medication, especially antihypertensives. Low-dose aspirin should be considered to decrease the risk of superimposed pre-eclampsia.

Renal transplant recipients

Women are advised to wait for 1–2 years after transplantation before trying to conceive. This gives time for the graft function to stabilize on the lowest doses of immunosuppressives. Living related donor kidney transplants have better recipient survival rates. Outcomes are as for other chronic renal disease patients.

Acute renal failure

As outside pregnancy, the causes can be broadly subdivided into:

Prerenal, e.g. maternal sepsis, blood loss

Renal, e.g. acute tubular necrosis due to pre-eclampsia and associated disorders (especially Haemolysis, Elevated Liver enzymes, and Low Platelets—HELLP) or drugs such as non-steroidal anti-inflammatories

Post-renal, e.g. ureteric damage or obstruction.

Treatment depends on the underlying cause. Care must be taken not to fluid-overload the patient. Acute tubular necrosis is usually reversible; however, temporary dialysis may be necessary.

Further reading

Nelson-Piercy C (2010). Renal disease. In *Handbook of obstetric medicine*, 4th edn, Chapter 10, pp. 176–92. Informa Healthcare, London.

Williams D (2006). Renal disorders. In DK James, PJ Steer, CP Weiner, B Gonik, eds. *High risk pregnancy: management options*, 3rd edn, pp. 1098–124. Saunders Elsevier, UK.

Key information for the effects of pregnancy on chronic renal impairment

Degree of renal impairment	Mild (creatinine <125 mmol/L)	Moderate (creatinine <170 mmol/L)	Severe (creatinine <220 mmol/L)	Creatinine >220 mmol/L
Loss of function	2%	40%	65%	75%
Post-partum deterioration	20%	50%	60%	
End-stage renal failure	2%	33%	40%	

Key information for the effects of the degree of chronic renal impairment on pregnancy outcome

Degree of renal impairment	Mild (creatinine <125 mmol/L)	Moderate (creatinine 125–249 mmol/L)	Severe (creatinine >250 mmol/L)
Maternal complications, e.g. pre-eclampsia	25%	50%	85%
IUGR		30%	60%
Preterm delivery		55%	70%
Successful outcome	85–95%	60–90%	20–30%

Cardiac disease and pregnancy

Key learning points

Cardiac disease is the leading cause of maternal death, and the majority is caused by acquired, not congenital, heart disease

Multidisciplinary care and communication are essential

An individual risk assessment should be made for each patient and should include the effect of:

Genetics

Teratogenicity and pharmacokinetics of drugs

Physiology of pregnancy, labour, and puerperium

Abnormalities of pregnancy, labour, and puerperium which might occur.

Introduction

Maternal mortality from cardiac disease, although uncommon, is the leading cause of maternal death in the UK, and its incidence is increasing. The rise associated with acquired heart disease is due to the changing demographics of the pregnant population (increasing age and obesity). Ischaemic heart disease, aortic dissection, and peripartum cardiomyopathy are the most important acquired conditions and occur in previously asymptomatic individuals.

Deaths from congenital heart disease (CHD) are reducing, despite the increase in women delivering with corrected CHD. Undiagnosed CHD is a particular risk in migrant women—a thorough cardiological assessment of these women at booking is essential.

Physiological changes in pregnancy

- Stroke volume increases, maximum at 20 weeks
- Pulse rate increases
- Cardiac output increases, maximum at 20–34 weeks
- Smooth muscle relaxation results in BP dropping in early and mid-pregnancy and rising in late pregnancy
- Labour increases cardiac output further
- Post-natal relief of inferior vena cava (IVC) compression and autotransfusion of blood from within the uterus results in immediate further increases in circulating volume.

The ability to tolerate these changes must be considered for each individual woman with heart disease and an individual risk assessment made. The increase in circulating volume can cause decompensation in women with, e.g. obstructive valve lesions, pulmonary hypertension, dilated cardiomyopathy, and impaired ventricular function.

The reduced systemic vascular resistance reduces the afterload and hence may improve left-to-right shunts, but right-to-left shunts may worsen. For example, Eisenmenger's syndrome carries a 50% mortality rate. Consideration must also be given to teratogenicity of drug therapy and the genetic risk of CHD.

Principles of care

- Care should be multidisciplinary with cardiologist, obstetrician, and obstetric anaesthetist, each with expertise in managing cardiological problems in pregnancy. This may require referral to a tertiary centre
- Prior to pregnancy, the risks and implications of a pregnancy should be discussed with the woman, in order for her to make a decision regarding conception. Good contraception should be advised for those women for whom pregnancy is contraindicated
- Good communication and written management plans are essential. An individual risk assessment plan should be revised and communicated as pregnancy progresses
- Fetal echocardiography should be offered in view of the increased risk of CHD in the fetus

- Place, timing, and mode of delivery should be planned. An epidural is frequently recommended to minimize cardiovascular stress. Consideration should be given to the effects of drugs and fluids often used in labour (e.g. prostaglandins, oxytocin, IV fluids), the advisability of an assisted delivery to avoid bearing down or a C/S, PPH prophylaxis, post-natal anticoagulation, and post-natal care.

Major acquired cardiac conditions

Peripartum cardiomyopathy

- Unknown aetiology
- Causes 20% of cardiac maternal deaths in the UK
- Heart failure in the absence of a known cause, with onset between the last month of pregnancy and up to 5 months post-partum
- Presents with symptoms and signs of heart failure ± systemic emboli
- If cardiac function does not normalize, 50% worsen and 25% risk death in further pregnancies
- If cardiac function normalizes, risk of recurrence in subsequent pregnancies.

Aortic dissection

- Consider in any woman with severe central chest pain, particularly radiating through to back
- Associated with systolic hypertension
- More common with Marfan's syndrome, Ehlers–Danlos syndrome, and aortopathy
- Normal CXR does not exclude diagnosis
- Diagnose with CT, MRI, or echocardiography
- Urgent surgical management is essential.

Myocardial infarction

- Incidence increasing as women delay childbearing
- Mortality rate of about 5%
- Arteriosclerosis is the most common cause, but coronary artery dissection is common in pregnancy
- Not usually preceded by angina
- Treatment as for non pregnant. Thrombolysis, if used, can be associated with bleeding.

Further reading

European Society of Cardiology (2011). *Cardiovascular diseases during pregnancy (management of)*. ESC clinical practice guidelines. Available at: <http://www.escardio.org/guidelines-surveys/esc-guidelines/Pages/cardiovascular-diseases-during-pregnancy.aspx>.

Royal College of Obstetricians and Gynaecologists (2011). *Cardiac disease and pregnancy (Good practice No. 13)*. Available at: <http://www.rcog.org.uk/files/rcog-corp/GoodPractice13CardiacDiseaseandPregnancy.pdf>.

Care pathway for cardiac disease and pregnancy

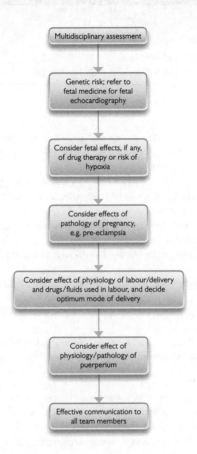

Multidisciplinary assessment

↓

Genetic risk; refer to fetal medicine for fetal echocardiography

↓

Consider fetal effects, if any, of drug therapy or risk of hypoxia

↓

Consider effects of pathology of pregnancy, e.g. pre-eclampsia

↓

Consider effect of physiology of labour/delivery and drugs/fluids used in labour, and decide optimum mode of delivery

↓

Consider effect of physiology/pathology of puerperium

↓

Effective communication to all team members

Anaemia in pregnancy

Key learning points

Physiology of haematological changes in pregnancy

Antenatal management of severe anaemia

Careful peripartum management to reduce risk of haemorrhage.

Aetiology

- Physiological relative reduction in Hb concentration and haematocrit in pregnancy
- Increase in plasma volume is relatively greater than of red cell mass (physiological anaemia)
- Effect increases with advancing gestation
- BUT pathological anaemia should not be overlooked. Significant anaemia (Hb <10.5 g/dL), particularly at booking, is less likely to be physiological, and other causes should be sought
- Erythrocyte size should be checked
- Haemoglobinopathies should be excluded, particularly in ethnically susceptible women (assessed as part of the screening tests taken at booking)
- Thalassaemia/sickle cell disease should be managed jointly with a haematologist and offered prenatal diagnostic testing
- In the absence of haemoglobinopathies, B12 and folate deficiencies should be excluded and iron deficiency assessed
- Chronic disease or malnutrition (particularly with coexisting hyperemesis gravidarum) may lead to an iron deficiency
- Treat anaemia in pregnancy—it is associated with an increase in adverse obstetric events, including PPH and infection. Effective antenatal treatment also reduces the need for peripartum blood transfusion.

Antenatal management

- Pregnant women obtain virtually all necessary vitamins and minerals from a healthy, balanced diet— except folic acid (in the first trimester, reducing the risk of NTDs) and, for some, iron. It is not clear why some women develop iron deficiency, even with good diet
- The mainstay of treatment of iron deficiency is supplemental iron. Oral iron can be unpleasant to take, with GI side effects (related to dose)—try different formulations such as syrups (iron is toxic in overdosage)
- It can take weeks or months to correct iron deficiency; therefore, treatment should be started as soon as the diagnosis is made
- Appropriate iron supplementation reduces the incidence of anaemia in pregnancy by about 40%
- Parenteral irons (usually IV sucrose or dextran, or occasionally IM) are effective when oral preparations are not tolerated (British National Formulary (BNF) advises facilities for cardiopulmonary resuscitation (CPR) should be available when giving IV treatment—small incidence of anaphylaxis).

Peripartum management

- Women giving birth with significant iron-deficient anaemia are at increased risk of adverse obstetric outcomes
- Women with severe anaemia in the third trimester may benefit from blood transfusion before birth to improve haematocrit rapidly
- IV access and crossmatching in labour are advisable
- There is little evidence to determine the safety of erythropoietin in pregnancy, and it is rarely used at present
- Some women find blood transfusion unacceptable for religious or other reasons. This can pose ethical and legal challenges for obstetricians, particularly in life-threatening situations. These women should be

counselled antenatally and have individualized care plans to deal with anaemia and to agree treatment in the event of major haemorrhage.

Further reading

British Medical Association; Royal Pharmaceutical Society (2011). *British National Formulary*. Issue 62, September 2011. BMJ Group and Pharmaceutical Press, London.

Dodd JM, Dare MR, Middleton P (2004). Treatment for women with postpartum iron deficiency anaemia. *Cochrane Database of Systematic Reviews*, **4**, CD004222.

Reveiz L, Gyte GML, Cuervo LG, Casasbuenas A (2011). Treatments for iron-deficiency anaemia in pregnancy. *Cochrane Database of Systematic Reviews*, **10**, CD003094.

Algorithm for anaemia in pregnancy

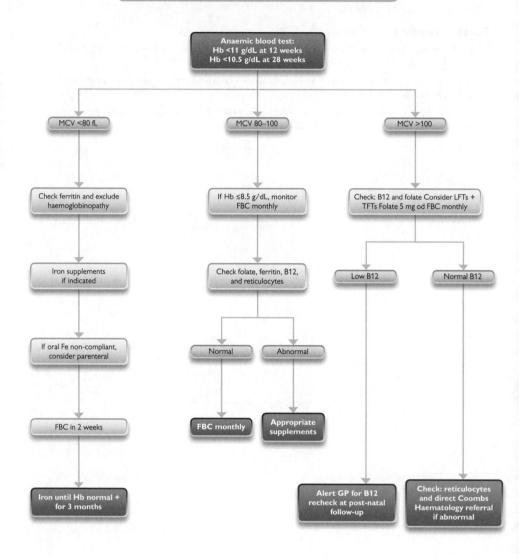

Jaundice

> ## Key learning points
> Causes of jaundice in pregnancy
> Effect of jaundice on mother and fetus
> Clinical assessment
> Principles of management.

Introduction

Jaundice complicates one in 1500 pregnancies. Viral hepatitis accounts for the majority of cases, while obstetric cholestasis, gallstones, hyperemesis gravidarum, acute fatty liver, and hypertensive diseases of pregnancy form other important aetiologies. Physiological changes of pregnancy are associated with mild cholestasis and elevated serum levels of alkaline phosphatase, fibrinogen, and most clotting factors. Serum protein concentrations and levels of serum transaminases are slightly reduced in normal pregnancy, while bilirubin levels do not show a significant change.

History

- Recent travel
- Past and current medical or surgical illnesses
- Drugs, substance abuse, and blood product transfusion
- Family history of jaundice or liver disease
- Symptoms of pruritus, abdominal pain, nausea, vomiting, fever
- Colour and consistency of stools.

Clinical examination

- Cutaneous manifestations of liver disease, palmar erythema, and spider naevi (present in 60% of normal pregnant women)
- Degree of jaundice
- Hydration status
- Consciousness level
- Cardiovascular stability
- Ecchymoses
- Ascites
- Hepatosplenomegaly
- Flapping tremors
- Obstetric examination and assessment of fetal well-being.

Management

- Hospitalization may be necessary for investigation and monitoring.
- Investigations
  - FBC
  - Urea and electrolytes (U + Es)
  - Liver function tests (LFTs)
  - Bile salts
  - Coagulation profile
  - Viral hepatitis screen
  - Autoimmune screen (anti-mitochondrial and anti-smooth muscle antibodies)
  - Urine analysis
  - USS of the liver and biliary tract should be performed
  - Liver biopsy if indicated (coagulation screen should be normal).

Multidisciplinary management should be instituted to identify and treat the aetiology as well as carry out supportive therapy with maintenance of hydration and nutrition, correction of electrolyte disturbances/coagulopathy, and control of blood glucose levels. Intensive care with ventilatory support may become necessary in severe cases. Depending on the aetiology and severity of the disease, it may be necessary to expedite delivery, even though the fetus may be premature.

Liver diseases peculiar to pregnancy

1. Hyperemesis gravidarum—associated with raised liver transaminases

2. Severe pre-eclampsia can lead to liver infarction, subcapsular haemorrhages, and/or HELLP syndrome. The patient presents with epigastric pain, nausea, vomiting, and hepatic tenderness, besides raised BP and proteinuria. Treatment is by delivery of the fetus, correction of coagulopathy, and supportive management

3. Intrahepatic cholestasis of pregnancy (obstetric cholestasis)—this presents with pruritus (without a skin rash) which involves trunk and limbs. It usually presents in third trimester and resolves spontaneously after delivery. It is a diagnosis of exclusion, and blood tests reveal raised bile acids and abnormal LFTs. Vitamin K supplementation, ursodeoxycholic acid, and regular fetal surveillance are important, and delivery is recommended by 37–38 weeks to avoid risk of stillbirth. Up to 45% of cases recur in subsequent pregnancies and with the use of combined oral contraceptive pills

4. Acute fatty liver of pregnancy—affects 1 in 10 000 pregnancies. It usually presents in third trimester and is associated with multiple pregnancy, a male fetus, and mild pre-eclampsia. Maternal and fetal mortality with this condition ranges from 18 to 23%. Clinical features include abdominal pain, nausea and vomiting, jaundice, headache, fever, confusion, and coma. Symptoms can progress rapidly to fulminant liver failure, disseminated intravascular coagulation (DIC), and renal failure. Hypoglycaemia is common. Investigations may reveal marked hyperuricaemia and fatty liver on ultrasound. These women should receive multidisciplinary care in HDU/ITU settings. Treatment of hypoglycaemia, vitamin K, fresh frozen plasma, strict fluid balance, and BP control form the mainstay of management. Stabilization of the woman should be followed by delivery. Although most women recover fully post-partum, some with fulminant hepatic failure may need transfer to a specialist liver unit.

Liver diseases incidental to pregnancy

1. Acute viral hepatitis—may be caused by viruses such as hepatitis A, B, C, D and E, herpes simplex, CMV, Epstein–Barr, or varicella zoster. Hepatitis A is usually a self-limiting illness, whilst hepatitis E tends to run a more severe course during pregnancy. Hepatitis during pregnancy increases the risk of preterm delivery. In case of hepatitis B, the neonate of an infected mother requires immunoprophylaxis at birth

2. Autoimmune hepatitis (chronic active hepatitis, primary biliary cirrhosis, sclerosing cholangitis)

3. Gall bladder calculi—acute cholecystitis is managed conservatively with hydration, analgesia, antiemetics, and antibiotics. Cholecystectomy may be indicated in patients with recurrent biliary colic or obstructive cholelithiasis

4. Congenital hyperbilirubinaemia—Gilbert's, Dubin–Johnson, and Rotor syndromes. Pregnancy may aggravate jaundice. Fetal outcome is usually good

5. Cirrhosis

6. Drug-induced hepatotoxicity

7. Malignancy

8. Other conditions—Budd–Chiari syndrome, Wilson's disease.

In utero exposure to elevated levels of unconjugated bilirubin does not necessarily result in fetal neurological or developmental abnormality; however, the risk depends on the integrity of the blood-brain barrier. Perinatal mortality rate is increased in cases of acute fatty liver, hypertensive diseases of pregnancy, and primary biliary cirrhosis.

Care pathway for jaundice

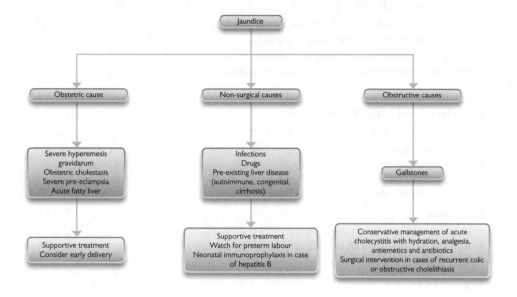

Jaundice

Obstetric cause

Severe hyperemesis gravidarum
Obstetric cholestasis
Severe pre-eclampsia
Acute fatty liver

Supportive treatment
Consider early delivery

Non-surgical causes

Infections
Drugs
Pre-existing liver disease
(autoimmune, congenital, cirrhosis)

Supportive treatment
Watch for preterm labour
Neonatal immunoprophylaxis in case of hepatitis B

Obstructive causes

Gallstones

Conservative management of acute cholecystitis with hydration, analgesia, antiemetics and antibiotics
Surgical intervention in cases of recurrent colic or obstructive cholelithiasis

Hypertension in pregnancy

Key learning points

Definition and classification of hypertension in pregnancy

Antenatal prediction and detection of hypertension

Management of severe hypertension in pregnancy

Effects of proteinuric hypertension on fetus and mother.

Definition and classification

A systolic BP ≥140 mmHg and/or a diastolic BP ≥90 mmHg.

- **Chronic hypertension**—present at booking or prior to 20 weeks, can be essential or secondary
- **Gestational hypertension**—new hypertension without proteinuria, presenting after 20 weeks
- **Pre-eclampsia**—new hypertension with proteinuria, presenting after 20 weeks
- **Pre-eclampsia superimposed on chronic hypertension**.

Incidence

- 20% of women are hypertensive at some stage of their pregnancy
- 5–10% of primigravid and 2% of multigravid women develop pre-eclampsia
- Ten to 25% of women with chronic hypertension develop superimposed pre-eclampsia.

Pre-eclampsia

A syndrome characterized by multisystem organ dysfunction. It leads to both maternal and fetal consequences.

Maternal risks—eclampsia (seizures), stroke, DIC, renal failure, liver failure or rupture, operative delivery, death.

Fetal risks—growth restriction, placental abruption, consequences of prematurity, perinatal death.

Risk factors

- Primigravida
- Increased maternal age
- Family history
- New partner
- Obesity
- Diabetes
- Chronic hypertension
- Autoimmune disease, e.g. antiphospholipid syndrome (APS), systemic lupus erythematosus (SLE)
- Renal disease
- Multiple pregnancy
- Previous pregnancy complicated by hypertension/pre-eclampsia.

Symptoms and signs of pre-eclampsia

Headache, visual disturbance, vomiting, oedema, epigastric pain, confusion.

Raised BP, proteinuria (protein:creatinine ratio >30 mg/mmol or 24-h protein >0.3 g/24 h), hyperreflexia, clonus, palpates small for dates.

Management

Pre-pregnancy

Offer high-risk women 75 mg aspirin daily from 12 weeks' gestation to delivery.

Optimize control of chronic hypertension prior to pregnancy.

Review antihypertensives and alter, if necessary, e.g. stop angiotensin-converting enzyme (ACE) inhibitors due to risk of congenital abnormalities.

Antenatal

Chronic hypertension—aim for BP <150/100 mmHg.

Ultrasound for fetal growth, liquor volume, and Doppler at 28–30 and 32–34 weeks. Observe for superimposed pre-eclampsia closely. Advise women to report any symptoms. If stable, do not deliver prior to 37 weeks.

If secondary chronic hypertension, will require specialist care and individualized management.

Gestational hypertension—review in secondary care. Test for proteinuria, renal and liver function, FBC ± growth scan.

Mild hypertension—BP 140/90–149/99 mmHg; observe closely as outpatient. Do not treat hypertension.

Moderate hypertension—BP 150/100–159/109 mmHg; commence antihypertensives, and manage as an outpatient.

Severe hypertension—BP >160/110 mmHg; commence antihypertensives, and observe as an inpatient. Observe for signs of pre-eclampsia. If BP stable, do not offer delivery before 37 weeks.

Pre-eclampsia—the ultimate 'cure' for pre-eclampsia is delivery of the baby and placenta.

Obviously, gestation and severity of the condition impact management.

Mild hypertension—do not treat. Check BP four times a day. Check FBC, renal and liver functions twice weekly.

Moderate hypertension—commence antihypertensives. Check BP four times a day, and FBC, renal and liver functions three times a week.

Severe hypertension—consider transfer to critical care ± seizure prevention with magnesium sulfate. Commence antihypertensives to keep BP <150/80–100 mmHg

If delivery required, consult with anaesthetic and neonatal staff, depending on severity and gestation.

If <34/40, give corticosteroids.

If over 37/40, NICE recommends delivery within 24–48 h of diagnosis of pre-eclampsia.

Medication

Labetalol is recommended as first-line treatment
Alternatives include methyldopa and nifedipine
For severe pre-eclampsia, IV labetalol or hydralazine may be needed.

Intrapartum

Hourly BP measurement
Fluid balance
Fetal monitoring
If BP stable, operative delivery only for obstetric indication.

Post-partum

Long-term management of chronic hypertension
If gestational hypertension or pre-eclampsia, observe BP closely for 24–48 h
Wean off antihypertensives gradually.

Advise woman on the risk of recurrence in future pregnancies:

If gestational hypertension, then 16–50% risk of recurrence and up to 7% risk of pre-eclampsia
If pre-eclampsia, then 1 in 6 chance of recurrence
If severe pre-eclampsia needing delivery before 34 weeks, then 25% chance of recurrence or 50% if delivery before 28 weeks.

All are associated with the development of hypertension and its complications later in life.

Further reading

Goh J and Flynn M (2004). *Examination obstetrics & gynaecology*, 2nd edn. Elsevier Australia, Marrickville.

National Institute for Health and Clinical Excellence (2010). *Hypertension in pregnancy: the management of hypertensive disorders during pregnancy*. NICE clinical guideline 107. Available at: <http://www.nice.org.uk/nicemedia/live/13098/50418/50418.pdf>.

Algorithm for the treatment of hypertension in pregnancy

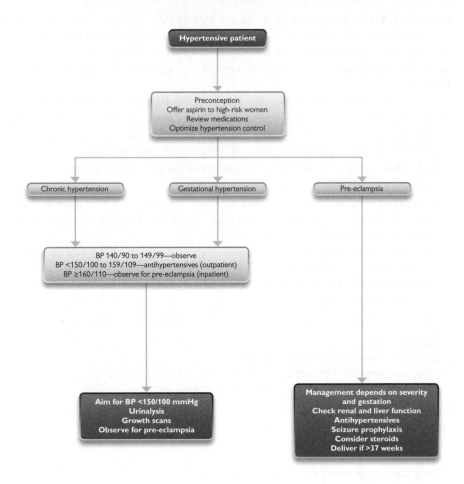

Hypertensive patient

Preconception
Offer aspirin to high-risk women
Review medications
Optimize hypertension control

| Chronic hypertension | Gestational hypertension | Pre-eclampsia |

BP 140/90 to 149/99—observe
BP <150/100 to 159/109—antihypertensives (outpatient)
BP ≥160/110—observe for pre-eclampsia (inpatient)

Aim for BP <150/100 mmHg
Urinalysis
Growth scans
Observe for pre-eclampsia

Management depends on severity
and gestation
Check renal and liver function
Antihypertensives
Seizure prophylaxis
Consider steroids
Deliver if >37 weeks

Asthma in pregnancy

Key learning points

Physiological changes to the respiratory tract in pregnancy

Symptoms, signs, and triggers of attacks

Effect of treatment regimes on mother and fetus during pregnancy

Limited available data for newer drugs in pregnancy.

Background

The symptom of breathlessness is common in pregnancy. This physiological change is progesterone-mediated and is due to significant increases in oxygen demand. Pregnant women increase their minute ventilation by nearly 50% by increasing the volume of each breath, rather than by increasing their respiratory rate. Diaphragmatic splinting due to the enlarged uterus also occurs in the third trimester. Peak expiratory flow rate (PEFR) and forced expiratory volume in 1 second (FEV1) remain unaltered in normal pregnancy.

It can be difficult to distinguish normal physiological changes from asthma. Asthma is the commonest medical illness to complicate pregnancy, affecting up to 7% of women of childbearing age.

Symptoms

- Breathlessness
- Wheezy breathing
- Cough
- Chest tightness
- Often worse at night and in the early morning
- Trigger factors, e.g. pollen, upper respiratory tract infection.

Clinical signs are often absent unless during an acute attack. Then, increased respiratory rate, inability to complete sentences, wheeze, use of accessory muscles, and tachycardia may all be noted.

The pathogenesis of asthma is reversible bronchoconstriction. This is assessed using a peak flow meter and measuring the decreased PEFR and FEV1. These values should improve following inhalation of a β_2 sympathomimetic bronchodilator.

Mild asthma in pregnancy

Most patients will not run into problems in pregnancy, provided they continue to use their pre-pregnancy medication and this was adequate. Patients are often reluctant to take medication, especially in the first trimester, but they must be encouraged to do so. Some will experience post-natal deterioration of symptoms. Prevention, rather than treatment of acute attacks, should be the emphasis. It is wise to check the woman's inhaler technique, since a 'breath-activated spacer' may be helpful.

Severe asthma in pregnancy

Women with severe asthma and poorly controlled asthmatics are more likely to experience a deterioration in their respiratory function in pregnancy. Ideally, preconception stabilization/escalation of medication makes pregnancy management easier. These patients often have acute exacerbations in the third trimester due to diaphragmatic splinting. If the mother is chronically or intermittently hypoxaemic, the fetus may be growth-restricted and serial growth scans are necessary. Occasionally, early delivery is necessary on fetal/ maternal grounds. A multidisciplinary team should be involved in such difficult decisions.

It is unusual to have acute asthma attacks in labour due to increased endogenous steroids. Early epidural is preferable in severe asthmatic patients in labour due to the decreased risk of atelectasis, should emergency surgery be necessary.

Prophylactic management of asthma

Management follows a stepwise approach (British Thoracic Society/Scottish Intercollegiate Guidelines Network). This is summarized in the Care Pathway. There are no major differences from the management of asthma outside pregnancy. All the drugs used appear to be safe in pregnancy and during lactation. The leukotriene receptor antagonists, e.g. montelukast, are relatively new agents, and there are limited available data in pregnancy. The current advice is neither to stop them in pregnancy nor to start them.

It is important to remember that, if the woman is on regular oral steroids antenatally, she is at risk of gestational diabetes mellitus and she should be tested for this at 28 weeks' gestation unless indicated earlier. She will also require regular IV hydrocortisone in labour due to the 'stress' of labour and her suppressed hypothalamic-pituitary axis.

Asthmatics may be 'sensitive' to aspirin, even in low doses. They may also respond badly to β-blockers. Prostaglandin $F_{2\alpha}$ and ergot alkaloids for the management of the third stage of labour can also cause bronchospasm and should be avoided, if possible.

Emergency management of acute attacks

The management is the same as outside pregnancy:

- High-flow oxygen
- Nebulized $β_2$ agonists
- Nebulized ipratropium bromide
- IV or oral steroids
- IV rehydration.

Further treatment should involve respiratory physicians and intensivists.

Poor psychosocial factors can increase the risk of death from asthma. The incidence of death due to asthma in pregnancy (an 'indirect' cause of death) has remained unchanged over recent years (4–5 cases per year).

Breastfeeding

The risk of atopy in a child of an asthmatic mother is about 1 in 10 or 1 in 3 if both parents are atopic. There is some evidence that breastfeeding may decrease this risk. This may be a result of the delay in the introduction of cow's milk protein.

Further reading

British Thoracic Society and Scottish Intercollegiate Guideline Network (2011). British Guideline in Asthma Management: a national clinical guideline. Thorax, 58 (Suppl) or, https://www.brit-thoracic.org.uk/document-library/clinical-information/asthma/btssign-guideline-on-the-management-of-asthma/, Sections 7.4–7.8, pp. 85–90.

Nelson-Piercy C (2010). Respiratory disease. In *Handbook of obstetric medicine*, 4th edn, Chapter 4, pp. 57–78. Informa Healthcare, London.

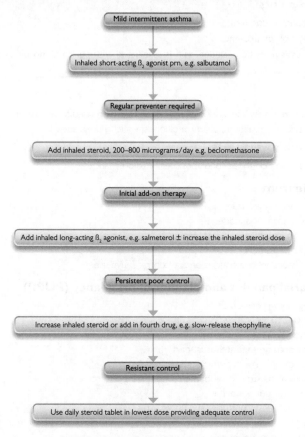

Care pathway for asthma in pregnancy

Mild intermittent asthma

↓

Inhaled short-acting ß₂ agonist prn, e.g. salbutamol

↓

Regular preventer required

↓

Add inhaled steroid, 200–800 micrograms/day e.g. beclomethasone

↓

Initial add-on therapy

↓

Add inhaled long-acting ß₂ agonist, e.g. salmeterol ± increase the inhaled steroid dose

↓

Persistent poor control

↓

Increase inhaled steroid or add in fourth drug, e.g. slow-release theophylline

↓

Resistant control

↓

Use daily steroid tablet in lowest dose providing adequate control

Data from British Thoracic Society, Scottish Intercollegiate Guideline Network 2011 British Guideline in Asthma Management: a national clinical guideline. Thorax, 58 (Suppl). <http://www.brit-thoracic.org.uk/Portals/0/Guidelines/AsthmaGuidelines/sign101%20Jan%202012.pdf>

Pruritus in pregnancy

Key learning points

Pruritus in pregnancy is common

Rash may, or may not, be present

Obstetric cholestasis must be excluded, as it is associated with perinatal morbidity and mortality.

Introduction

Pruritus (itchiness) in pregnancy affects 17% of women and can be related to pre-existing skin conditions, such as eczema or psoriasis, drug reactions, or to conditions specific to pregnancy.

Pruritus can occur with or without a rash.

This chapter will focus only on those conditions specific to pregnancy.

Pruritus gravidarum

- Usually occurs in early pregnancy
- Not associated with rash or jaundice
- Treat with topical antipruritics ± antihistamines
- Settles rapidly post-partum
- Can recur with subsequent pregnancies or oral contraceptive use.

Pruritic urticarial papules and plaques of pregnancy (PUPP)

- Commonest pregnancy-specific rash
- Incidence of 1/200–250 pregnancies
- Usually occurs after 35 weeks' gestation
- Up to 15% initially occur immediately post-partum
- Three-quarters of cases occur in primiparous women
- Papules and plaques along striae on abdomen, with sparing of umbilicus
- Small vesicles can occur but not bullae
- Can spread to thighs, breasts, buttocks, and upper arms
- Pathogenesis unknown but may be related to skin distension, as more common in multiple gestations and pregnancies with excessive weight gain
- Resolves rapidly after delivery
- No fetal risks
- Can be associated with maternal hypertension
- Treat with 1% aqueous menthol cream, topical steroids ± antihistamines
- Recurrence is rare and usually mild.

Pemphigoid (herpes) gestationis

- Incidence 1/1700–1/50 000 pregnancies
- Usually occurs in second or third trimester
- Can persist or flare post-partum
- Autoimmune aetiology
- Affects primiparous and multiparous women
- Pruritus may precede the rash which typically starts on and around umbilicus
- Erythematous papules and plaques are followed by vesicles and tense bullae
- Direct immunofluorescence shows C3 deposition in basement membrane
- Increased risk of IUGR and low birthweight
- As it is an autoimmune disease, up to 10% of newborns have a mild rash that resolves within weeks
- Treat with potent topical steroids or oral steroids ± sedative antihistamines

- Usually recurs in subsequent pregnancies, with earlier onset and greater severity
- May also recur with oral contraceptive use and/or menstruation
- Increased lifetime risk of Graves's disease.

Prurigo of pregnancy

- Incidence 1/300–1/450 pregnancies
- Begins in second or third trimester
- Pruritic excoriated red/brown papules on trunk and extensor surfaces of limbs
- Pruritus resolves after delivery, but papules can persist for months
- Aetiology unknown but associated with atopy
- Treat with topical steroids ± antihistamines
- No fetal risks
- Can recur in subsequent pregnancies.

Pruritic folliculitis of pregnancy

- Incidence unknown
- Mainly occurs in third trimester
- Acneiform, pruritic, follicular papules and pustules
- Widespread distribution
- Settles before delivery and not associated with post-partum flare
- ? form of hormone-induced acne
- Treat with topical 10% benzoyl peroxide, mild topical steroids ± antihistamines
- No associated fetal risks
- Risk of recurrence unknown.

Obstetric cholestasis

- Incidence ranges from 01. to 15.6%
- Occurs in second and third trimesters
- Pruritus and elevation of bile salts but **NO** rash
- Pruritus particularly affects palms and soles
- Pathogenesis unknown but genetic, hormonal, and environmental factors involved
- Oestrogens cause cholestasis. Obstetric cholestasis is commoner in multiple pregnancies when oestrogen levels are higher
- 30% of patients give a positive family history
- Seasonal variation in incidence and higher rates in certain countries, e.g. Chile, may indicate the involvement of environmental factors
- Less than 10% of patients suffer from jaundice. Dark urine, pale stools, and anorexia may be associated symptoms
- Raised bile salts ± elevated transaminases and bilirubin ± altered coagulation help to confirm diagnosis
- Liver ultrasound, viral serology (hepatitis A, B, and C, EBV, and CMV), and liver autoantibody screen should be considered
- Maternal risks—vitamin K deficiency, increased risk of PPH
- Fetal risks—intrapartum fetal heart rate (FHR) abnormalities
  - Spontaneous and iatrogenic preterm delivery
  - Meconium passage
  - Intrauterine death
  - Intracranial haemorrhage
- Level of serum bile acids may correlate with fetal risk, but maternal symptom severity does not
- Rate of intrauterine death difficult to determine, as management usually involves induction of labour at 37(+) weeks' gestation.

Management

- Once diagnosis made, counsel regarding possible risks to fetus and need for close surveillance
- Weekly LFTs
- Fetal monitoring with cardiotocographies (CTGs) and ultrasound for fetal growth, liquor volume, and umbilical artery Doppler
- Offer induction of labour at 37–38 weeks' gestation
- Counsel woman regarding risks associated with early induction, e.g. failure, neonatal unit admission, increased maternal morbidity, but unknown risk of stillbirth if pregnancy continues
- Continuous fetal monitoring in labour
- IM vitamin K to baby after delivery
- Ursodeoxycholic acid to reduce bile acid levels, relieve pruritus, and improve liver function
- Vitamin K, 10–20 mg daily, may reduce risk of maternal and fetal bleeding
- Antihistamines
- Pruritus usually resolves quickly post-partum
- Check liver function 10 days post-delivery to ensure normalized
- Risk of recurrence in future pregnancies is 90%
- Women should be advised to avoid oestrogen-containing medication.

Further reading

de Swiet M (2002). *Medical disorders in obstetric practice*, 4th edn. Blackwell Science Ltd, Oxford.

Kroumpouzoz G, Cohen LM (2001). Dermatoses of pregnancy. *Journal of the American Academy of Dermatology*, **45**, 1–19.

Nelson-Piercy C (2005). *Handbook of obstetric medicine*, 2nd edn. Taylor and Francis Group.

Pierson JC and Tam CC (2012). *Pruritic uticarial papules and plaques of pregnancy clinical presentation*. Available at: <http://emedicine.medscape.com/article/1123725-clinical>.

Royal College of Obstetricians and Gynaecologists (2011). *Obstetric cholestasis*. Green-top guideline No. 43. Available at: <http://www.rcog.org.uk/files/rcog-corp/GTG43obstetriccholestasis.pdf>.

Care pathways for pruritus in pregnancy

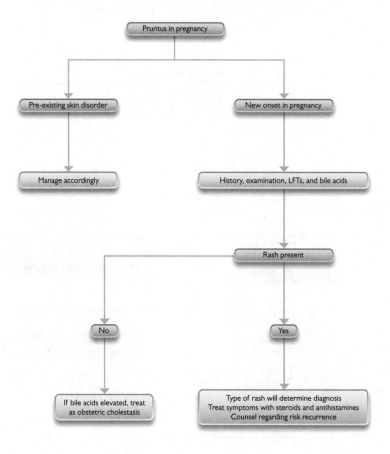

Care pathways for pruritus in pregnancy

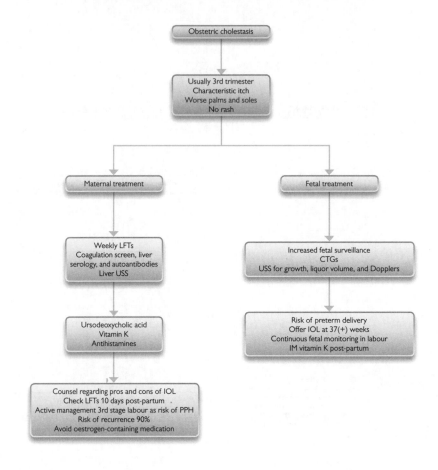

Obstetric cholestasis

Usually 3rd trimester
Characteristic itch
Worse palms and soles
No rash

Maternal treatment

Fetal treatment

Weekly LFTs
Coagulation screen, liver
serology, and autoantibodies
Liver USS

Increased fetal surveillance
CTGs
USS for growth, liquor volume, and Dopplers

Ursodeoxycholic acid
Vitamin K
Antihistamines

Risk of preterm delivery
Offer IOL at 37(+) weeks
Continuous fetal monitoring in labour
IM vitamin K post-partum

Counsel regarding pros and cons of IOL
Check LFTs 10 days post-partum
Active management 3rd stage labour as risk of PPH
Risk of recurrence 90%
Avoid oestrogen-containing medication

Liquor volume and fetal growth

Key learning points

Basic pathophysiology of liquor formation in normal and abnormal pregnancies
Distinguish between small-for-gestational-age (SGA) and IUGR fetuses
Principles of management includes identifying at-risk fetuses.

Pathophysiology

- Amniotic fluid is initially derived from the uteroplacental unit
- By 10 weeks, embryonic organs begin to excrete amniotic fluid
- By 22 weeks, fetal excretion and absorption mainly accounts for liquor volume
- Polyhydramnios is caused either by increased fetal excretion or impaired fetal absorption
- Oligohydramnios is caused by reduced excretion (or leakage through ruptured membranes) of liquor.

Reduced excretion may be prerenal or renal.
- Prerenal causes
  - Uteroplacental insufficiency (leading to reduced renal perfusion)
  - Congenital infection
  - Genetic syndromes or aneuploidy
- Renal causes
  - Bilateral renal agenesis
  - Polycystic kidneys or renal tract outflow obstruction
- Exclude spontaneous rupture of the amniotic membranes (SROM) as a cause
- Increased liquor production
  - May be seen with maternal diabetes due to hyperglycaemia
  - In a monochorionic twin (recipient) affected by TTTS, the fetus develops polyuria due to volume overload
  - Impaired fetal absorption occurs with defects of swallowing such as upper GI anomalies, diaphragmatic herniae, or thoracic masses
  - Neuromuscular anomalies can also diminish swallowing.

Fetal growth

- Growth is determined by genetic potential and substrate availability
- IUGR occurs when the fetus fails to grow to its genetic potential. Generally, the cause is uteroplacental insufficiency
- SGA occurs when the fetal size measures below a specific centile (e.g. 5th). The cause is usually constitutional
- Most IUGR fetuses are SGA. But not all SGA babies have IUGR
- Symmetrical IUGR occurs where the head, abdomen, and femur are all proportionately small
- Asymmetrical IUGR has small abdominal circumference and femur but more normal head circumference
- Ensure the pregnancy has been accurately dated to avoid inappropriate diagnoses of growth 'problems'.

Causes of growth restriction

Maternal causes

- Chronic disease (including renal, diabetes, autoimmune, and anaemia)
- Pregnancy-induced hypertensive disorders are strongly associated with IUGR
- Malnutrition is an important cause globally
- Toxins—typically cigarettes (especially cocaine and heroin), some medications.

Placental causes

- Uteroplacental insufficiency (UPI)
  - Maldevelopment of the uteroplacental vasculature
  - Smaller placental disc. Cord often eccentrically inserted
  - Fewer, narrower, straighter capillaries
  - Confined placental mosaicism—incidence of 1 in 70
- Fetal causes
  - Structural defects—including some cardiac defects, gastroschisis, single umbilical artery
  - Aneuploidy (reported as high as 1 in 5). Typically symmetrical
  - Congenital infection—including malaria, CMV, and toxoplasmosis
  - Genetic abnormalities—genomic imprinting, uniparental disomy (UPD)
  - Multiple pregnancy.

Excessive growth

- Fetal macrosomia occurs in poorly controlled diabetes—including gestational diabetes
- Excessive calorific intake associated with obesity
- Prader–Willi syndrome is a rare genetic cause of macrosomia—probably because of abnormal fetal insulin metabolism.

Investigations

Routine clinical examination may suggest that uterine size is inappropriate for gestation. Too high a fundal height may indicate polyhydramnios or macrosomia (or both), whereas oligohydramnios or IUGR may be revealed by finding a low fundal height. Ultrasound assessment of fetal biometry and amniotic fluid volume should be performed.

Polyhydramnios

- Detailed fetal anatomical survey, particularly of upper GI tract, movements, and swallowing
- Test for diabetes (GTT).

Oligohydramnios

- Exclude SROM
- Ultrasound assessment of fetal growth
- Doppler studies of fetal and maternal uterine blood flow
- Detailed fetal anatomical survey to include renal tract
- TORCH screen for infection
- Consider karyotype of the fetus and that of the placenta for mosaicism by placental biopsy.

Small for gestational age

- Detailed ultrasound of fetal anatomy, liquor volume, fetal and maternal Dopplers
- TORCH screen
- Consider amniocentesis/CVS (karyotype, mosaicism, and infection testing ± gene test, if indicated).

Large for gestational age (above 95th centile)

- Detailed anatomical survey, including amniotic fluid volume
- GTT.

Management

IUGR/oligohydramnios

- IUGR and oligohydramnios often go together
- There is no effective treatment at present
- In the most severe cases, the fetus may not attain a viable gestation or size

- Realistic counselling about the possible outcomes in the short and long term should be given. Dependent on results and prognosis (and jurisdiction), early delivery or termination of pregnancy may be offered
- Delivery may need to be expedited if there is maternal compromise: risk of hypertension/proteinuria (severe form: 'mirror syndrome')
- These pregnancies are at increased risk of serious complications, including abruption and stillbirth
- Steroids should be administered in the preterm period shortly before delivery to improve neonatal lung function
- Mode and timing of delivery will require careful planning with the parents and neonatal team
- If induction of labour, for continuous fetal monitoring
- If C/S for extremely low birthweight, may need to be classical incision
- Send placenta for histology
- Close maternal observation
- Post-natal counselling and plan for future pregnancies—modify risk factors; advise aspirin.

Macrosomia/polyhydramnios

- Often go together
- In diabetes, maximize control to prevent further excessive growth—liquor may normalize
- In severe macrosomia, the risk of difficult vaginal delivery should be anticipated (shoulder dystocia). Caesarean delivery may be considered
- Counsel about risks of complications, e.g. SROM/abruption/cord prolapse/malpresentation for polyhydramnios
- In gross polyhydramnios, therapeutic amnioreduction may alleviate maternal discomfort/respiratory embarrassment. Referral to fetal medicine may be appropriate.

Further reading

Dunk C, Huppertz B, Kingdom J (2009). Development of the placenta and its circulation. In CH Rodeck and MJ Whittle, eds. *Fetal medicine, basic science and clinical practice*, 2nd edn, pp. 69–96. Churchill Livingstone, London.

Peregrine E and Peebles D (2009). Fetal growth and growth restriction. In CH Rodeck and MJ Whittle, eds. *Fetal medicine, basic science and clinical practice*, 2nd edn, pp. 541–58. Churchill Livingstone, London.

Royal College of Obstetricians and Gynaecologists (2013). *The investigation and management of the small-for-gestational-age fetus*. Green-top guideline No. 31 (2nd edn). Available at: <http://www.rcog.org.uk/files/rcog-corp/22.3.13GTG31SGA.pdf>.

Algorithm for SGA/oligohydramnios

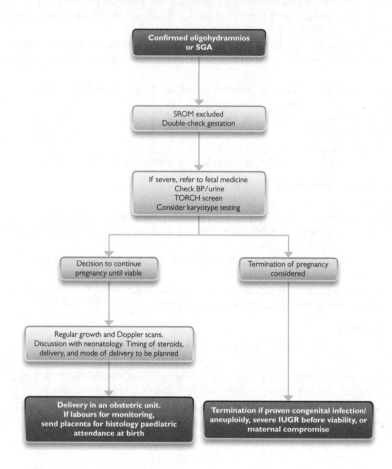

Confirmed oligohydramnios
or SGA

SROM excluded
Double-check gestation

If severe, refer to fetal medicine
Check BP/urine
TORCH screen
Consider karyotype testing

Decision to continue
pregnancy until viable

Termination of pregnancy
considered

Regular growth and Doppler scans.
Discussion with neonatology. Timing of steroids,
delivery, and mode of delivery to be planned

Delivery in an obstetric unit.
If labours for monitoring,
send placenta for histology paediatric
attendance at birth

Termination if proven congenital infection/
aneuploidy, severe IUGR before viability, or
maternal compromise

Algorithm for polyhydramnios/macrosomia

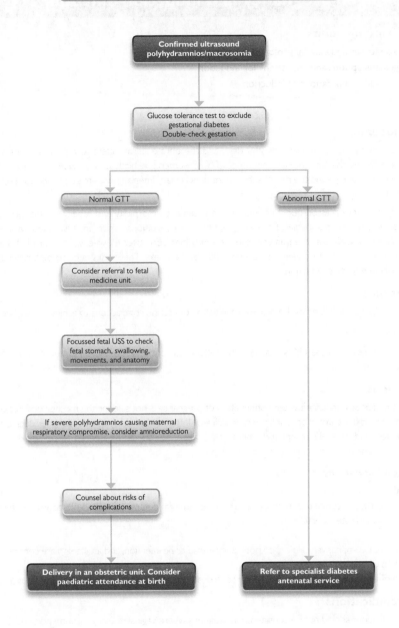

Confirmed ultrasound polyhydramnios/macrosomia

Glucose tolerance test to exclude gestational diabetes
Double-check gestation

Normal GTT

Abnormal GTT

Consider referral to fetal medicine unit

Focussed fetal USS to check fetal stomach, swallowing, movements, and anatomy

If severe polyhydramnios causing maternal respiratory compromise, consider amnioreduction

Counsel about risks of complications

Delivery in an obstetric unit. Consider paediatric attendance at birth

Refer to specialist diabetes antenatal service

Prolonged pregnancy and induction of labour

Key learning points

Risks to mother and baby of prolonged pregnancy

Management options and indications for induction

Methods and complications of induction.

Introduction

The median duration of pregnancy is 280 days, and the phrase 'term' refers to a pregnancy of 37 completed weeks onwards. Without intervention, 5–10% of women give birth after 42 weeks and are defined as 'post-term'. This figure—and the risk of subsequent unnecessary intervention—has been reduced by routine ultrasound scanning in early pregnancy.

Post-term pregnancy is associated with an increase in perinatal morbidity and otherwise unexplained mortality in structurally normal babies. For example, neonatal convulsions, which are associated with neonatal encephalopathy, are almost three times more likely in babies born after 41 weeks. The risk of stillbirth also rises from 2.1 per 1000 at 40 weeks to 2.6 per 1000 by 43 weeks. These risks need to be balanced against those of offering routine induction.

Definition

Induction of labour is defined as the process of initiation of uterine contractions to achieve vaginal delivery.

Incidence

One in five deliveries in the UK is induced. This reflects current policies, referral patterns, and sometimes maternal request.

Indications

Induction of labour is indicated when continuation of pregnancy is not safe for the mother or fetus or when both mother and fetus would benefit from early delivery. If the mother declines induction, her decision should be respected, and, after 42 completed weeks of gestation, she should be offered twice weekly CTG and ultrasound estimate of maximum amniotic fluid depth.

Common indications

Maternal

Medical or obstetric conditions, such as severe pre-eclampsia, deteriorating diabetic control, deteriorating renal function, indicate induction

Fetal

IUGR with fetal compromise, prolonged pregnancy, intrauterine infection, and fetal death are common causes of induction of labour.

Induction of labour for chorioamnionitis or uncontrolled diabetes benefits both mother and fetus.

Contraindications

Induction of labour should not be considered in situations where vaginal delivery is contraindicated. Examples include placenta praevia, cord presentation, active genital herpes, and previous uterine scar with midline or inverted T incision. Induction is contraindicated if labour threatens further fetal or maternal compromise.

Methods

Membrane sweeping

Membrane sweeping encourages the onset of spontaneous labour and reduces the need for formal induction of labour to prevent prolonged pregnancy. All women should be offered membrane sweeping at 41 weeks.

Pharmacological methods

Vaginal prostaglandin (PGE2) is the preferred method of induction of labour. It can be administered as gel, tablet, or controlled-release pessary. The following regimens are recommended by NICE:

One cycle of vaginal PGE2 tablets or gel: one dose, followed by a second dose after 6 h if labour is not established (up to a maximum of two doses)

One cycle of vaginal PGE2 controlled-release pessary: one dose over 24 h.

Vaginal misoprostol is not used for induction of labour in the UK but can be offered as method of induction to women who have IUFD or in the context of clinical trial.

Mifepristone should only be used as part of a treatment package to induce labour in women where fetal demise has occurred.

Mechanical methods

The available evidence has been reviewed by NICE, and it recommends that mechanical procedures (balloon catheters and laminaria tents) should not be used routinely for induction of labour. The evidence of efficacy of mechanical methods for induction of labour is not clear. They are not superior to prostaglandins.

Surgical methods

Artificial rupture of fetal membranes (ARM, amniotomy) requires a sufficiently dilated cervix for the introduction of a device with a hook to tear the membranes. In the presence of a favourable cervix, amniotomy is usually effective and may require subsequent oxytocin augmentation.

Process of induction of labour

The ease of induction of labour correlates well with the 'ripeness' of the cervix. This is assessed by the modified Bishop's score.

The Bishop's score (see Table 1) is a group of measurements taken from a vaginal examination and is based on the factors stated previously. The Bishop's score was modified by substituting the length of the cervix for the percentage of effacement.

A score of eight or more generally indicates that the cervix is ripe or 'favourable'—when there is a high chance of spontaneous labour or a good predicted response to interventions to induce labour. Whilst it is normally possible to induce labour with a favourable cervix, an unfavourable cervix can be made favourable by using vaginal prostaglandins.

Complications

The following complications can occur with induction of labour.

Uterine hyperstimulation

Hyperstimulation changes, with or without FHR, can occur in 1–5% of cases. Hyperstimulation is uncommon with low-dose PGE2 and can usually be reversed by β adrenergic therapy (single dose of terbutaline 250 micrograms intravenously over 5 min or subcutaneously).

Table 1 Modified Bishop's score

	Score			
	0	1	2	3
Cervical dilatation (cm)	0	1–2	3–4	>4
Cervical length (cm)	>4	2–4	1–2	<1
Cervical consistency	Firm	Medium	Soft	–
Cervical position	Posterior	Central	Anterior	
Station (cm to spines)	–3	–2	–1 to 0	+1/+2
	Above	Above	Above	Below spines

Reproduced with kind permission from Calder AA (1979) 'Management of unripe cervix' in MN JC Keirse, ABM Anderson (Eds), Human Parturition, pp. 201–217. Leiden: Leiden University Press.

Failed induction

Failed induction in the presence of an unfavourable cervix occurs in 15% of cases. When induction fails, the whole clinical situation should be reviewed, and subsequent management options should include a further attempt after a short delay to induce labour (clinical condition permitting) or to perform a C/S.

Cord prolapse

The incidence of cord prolapse is 0.1–0.5%, following membrane rupture. This complication is more likely to occur when the presenting fetal part is not well applied to the cervix.

Uterine rupture

Uterine rupture with induction of labour in nulliparous women is extremely rare but is a potential risk in multiparous women, particularly with previous Caesarean scar.

Outcome

Induction of labour is successful in the majority of cases. Generally, less than two-thirds of women will give birth without further intervention; about 15% will have instrumental births, and 22% will require emergency C/S.

Further reading

Calder AA (1979). Management of unripe cervix. In MJNC Keirse and ABM Anderson, eds. *Human parturition*, pp. 201–17. Leiden University Press, Leiden.

National Institute for Health and Clinical Excellence (2008). *Induction of labour*. NICE clinical guideline 70. Available at: <http://www.nice.org.uk/nicemedia/live/12012/41256/41256.pdf>.

Rayburn WF (1989). Prostaglandin E2 gel for cervical ripening and induction of labor: a critical analysis. *American Journal of Obstetrics and Gynecology*, **160**, 529–34.

Algorithm for prolonged pregnancy and induction of labour

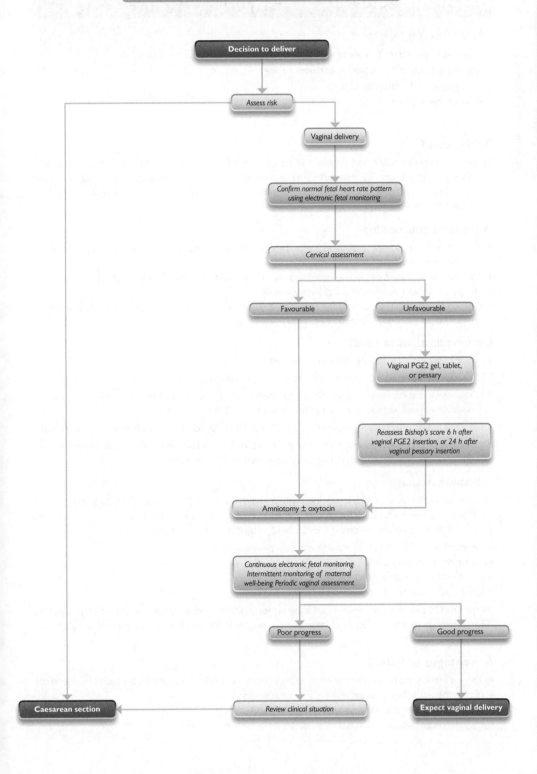

Decision to deliver

Assess risk

Vaginal delivery

Confirm normal fetal heart rate pattern using electronic fetal monitoring

Cervical assessment

Favourable

Unfavourable

Vaginal PGE2 gel, tablet, or pessary

Reassess Bishop's score 6 h after vaginal PGE2 insertion, or 24 h after vaginal pessary insertion

Amniotomy ± oxytocin

Continuous electronic fetal monitoring Intermittent monitoring of maternal well-being Periodic vaginal assessment

Poor progress

Good progress

Caesarean section

Review clinical situation

Expect vaginal delivery

Birth after Caesarean section

Key learning points

Advantages and disadvantages of vaginal birth after Caesarean section (C/S)

Support and advice to women in decision making

Managing vaginal birth after C/S

Risks of scar rupture.

Background

There is widespread public and professional concern about the increasing proportion of births by C/S. Increasing rates of primary C/S have led to greater percentages of the obstetric population having a history of prior C/S. Commonly, these women are offered vaginal birth after C/S (VBAC) or elective repeat C/S (ERCS) on the basis of 'maternal request' only.

Antenatal counselling

- Many obstetric units now have VBAC clinics. Their structure is varied, but their aim is to support and advise women who have had previous C/S
- The minimum requirement is that women are counselled, with a record of this in the notes
- The patient should also receive an information leaflet
- Women considering their options for birth after a single previous C/S should be informed that, overall, the chances of successful planned VBAC are 72–76%.

Contraindications to VBAC

1. Prior 'classical' C/S (vertical incision in upper part of uterus)

2. Previous J or inverted T-shaped incisions: some myomectomy incisions

3. Previous uterine dehiscence (disruption of the uterine muscle, with intact uterine serosa) or uterine rupture (with additional involvement of the serosa and adjacent structures)

4. More than two previous uncomplicated C/S (although the evidence for this is currently being reviewed).

A cautious approach is advised when considering planned VBAC with twin gestations, fetal macrosomia (albeit difficult to assess antenatally), and short interdelivery intervals (<12 months).

Intrapartum care

The predominant risk of VBAC is uterine rupture, which occurs in 1 in 200 such labours and can have extreme consequences for both the mother and fetus, even in a hospital setting. It is because of this risk we allow fully informed women to 'request' ERCS. Signs of uterine rupture include:

- An abnormal CTG—the most consistent finding in uterine rupture
- Cessation of contractions
- Severe and constant scar tenderness
- Others such as vaginal bleeding and bloodstained urine.

Women should be advised to deliver in a suitably equipped setting, and continuous electronic fetal monitoring (EFM) is strongly recommended. Epidural analgesia is not contraindicated, since 'scar pain' will break through this analgesia.

Advantages of VBAC

- There is a much decreased risk of transient tachypnoea of the newborn and respiratory problems after birth
- Mother/baby bonding is better with early skin-to-skin contact
- Breastfeeding rates are also improved.
- Early discharge home

- Start driving sooner
- Sense of achievement of having delivered vaginally.

Disadvantages of VBAC

- There is a slightly increased risk of blood transfusion and endometritis
- Small increased risk of birth-related perinatal death, but this is comparable to the risk for women having their first baby
- An additional risk of the infant developing hypoxic ischaemic encephalopathy.

Induction and augmentation

Of the two commonly used methods of induction of labour (IOL):

- Vaginal prostaglandins carry a 2.5% risk of scar rupture (vs 0.5% for spontaneous labour)
- Artificial rupture of the membranes (ARM) and oxytocin stimulation carry an intermediate risk
- For this reason, we offer IOL at term + 10 days, and perform regular cervical sweeps in the interim to encourage spontaneous labour.

Women need to be carefully counselled about these risks so they can make informed choices about IOL—it is not too late to opt for ERCS. Individual clinicians also tend to have personal viewpoints on this subject, particularly since this is an unlicensed use of prostaglandins. Some will not offer IOL at all.

- When oxytocin is being used for **augmentation**, there is a 1.5-fold increased risk of C/S. Great care must be taken by the obstetrician to ensure adequate progress is being made. The assumption is that genuine/relative cephalopelvic disproportion will increase the chance of scar rupture and should be avoided, if possible.

Further reading

Royal College of Obstetricians and Gynaecologists (2007). *Birth after previous Caesarean birth.* Green-top guideline No. 45. Available at: <http://www.rcog.org.uk/files/rcog-corp/GTG4511022011.pdf>.

Care pathway for birth after Caesarean (BAC)

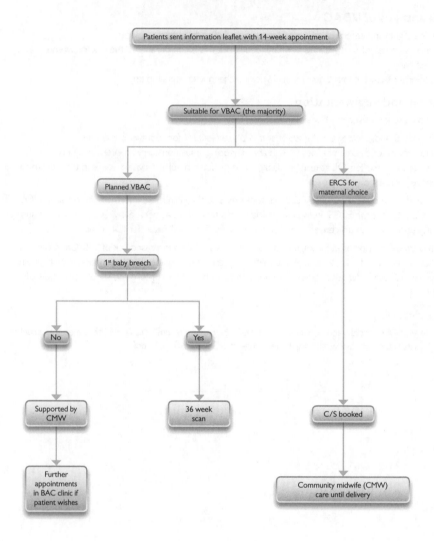

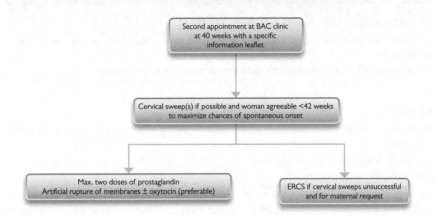

Care pathway for induction of labour visit in women planning BAC

Second appointment at BAC clinic at 40 weeks with a specific information leaflet

Cervical sweep(s) if possible and woman agreeable <42 weeks to maximize chances of spontaneous onset

Max. two doses of prostaglandin
Artificial rupture of membranes ± oxytocin (preferable)

ERCS if cervical sweeps unsuccessful and for maternal request

Diagnosis of labour

Key learning points

Onset of painful uterine contractions, along with progressive cervical dilatation, is essential for the diagnosis of labour

Accurate diagnosis of labour is essential to avoid intervention in the latent phase.

Introduction

Labour can be diagnosed from a combination of the patient's history and physical signs on examination. Labour is diagnosed by the combination of two features:

- Regular, painful uterine activity or contractions
- Progressive cervical changes.

Women admitted to hospital in the latent phase, and not yet in active labour, are more likely to receive medical intervention (e.g. oxytocin augmentation, EFM, C/S) than those admitted in active labour. Therefore, an incorrectly early diagnosis of labour has significant consequences. Between 30 and 45% of women admitted to labour wards in the UK and other developed countries are found not to be in active labour.

History

- Intermittent abdominal pain—strength, frequency, duration, and level of discomfort
- Tightening of uterus
- Bloodstained mucous discharge (or 'show')
- Sudden gush of water, with or without pain (rupture of membranes)
- Others
  - Backache
  - Nausea and vomiting
  - Diarrhoea, change of bowel habit.

Physical examination

Record general condition, pulse, BP, and urine dipstick.

Abdominal examination

- Note uterine contractions—frequency, duration
- Fundal height, lie, presentation, position, and station
- Fetal heart auscultation, using a Pinard or sonicaid, or EFM.

Vaginal examination

- Evidence of vaginal 'show'
- Evidence of membrane rupture
- Cervical changes
  - Dilatation: the increase in diameter of the cervical opening, measured in cm
  - Effacement
    - The progressive shortening and thinning of the cervix in labour
    - The length of the cervix is variable at the onset of labour (from a few mm to 3 cm), but, throughout labour, the length decreases steadily to a few mm
  - Initial cervical examination provides a baseline from which to assess progress.

Stages of labour

Labour is divided into three stages.

First stage

- Onset of labour to full dilatation of cervix, with a process of cervical effacement and dilatation

- Latent phase
  - Is the early part of the first stage of labour to 3–4 cm dilatation. It can last from a few hours to a few days
- Active phase
  - Cervix is between 4 and 10 cm dilated
  - Rate of cervical dilatation is usually 0.5–1 cm/h
  - Effacement is usually complete
  - Fetal descent through birth canal is complete.

Second stage

- From full dilatation of the cervix to delivery of the baby, by a process of descent of the fetus through the birth canal
- Early phase (non-expulsive)
  - Cervix is fully dilated
  - Fetal descent continues
  - No urge to push
- Late phase (expulsive)
  - Fetal part reaches the pelvic floor
  - Urge to push
  - Birth should be expected to take place by 3 h of the start of active second stage in nulliparous, and 2 h in multiparous, women.

Third stage

- From delivery of the baby until delivery of the placenta and membranes. It usually lasts no more than 30 min.

Differential diagnosis

- Braxton–Hicks contractions
- UTI, resulting in uterine irritability
- Prolonged latent phase of labour
- Bowel symptoms.

Further reading

Cheyne H, Hundley V, Dowding D, et al. (2008). Effects of algorithm for diagnosis of active labour: cluster randomised trial. *BMJ*, **337**, a2396.

Holmes P, Oppenheimer LW, Wen SW (2001). The relationship between cervical dilatation at initial presentation in labour and subsequent intervention. *British Journal of Obstetrics and Gynaecology*, **108**, 1120–4.

National Institute for Health and Clinical Excellence (2007). *Intrapartum care: care of healthy women and their babies during childbirth*. NICE clinical guideline 55. Available at: <http://www.nice.org.uk/nicemedia/pdf/IPCNICEguidance.pdf>.

Algorithm for the diagnosis of labour

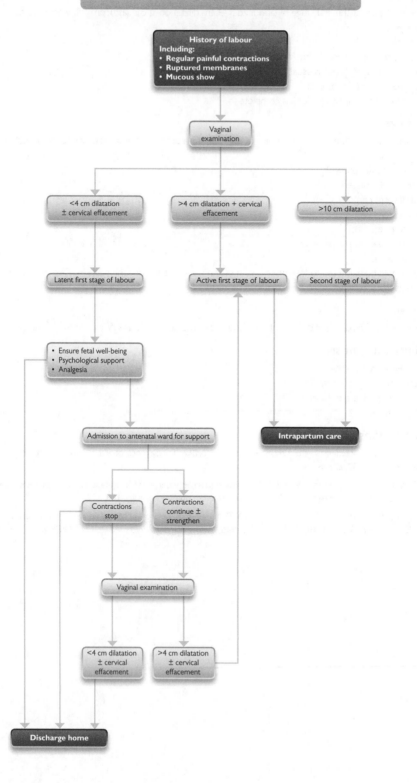

History of labour
Including:
- Regular painful contractions
- Ruptured membranes
- Mucous show

Vaginal examination

<4 cm dilatation ± cervical effacement

>4 cm dilatation + cervical effacement

>10 cm dilatation

Latent first stage of labour

Active first stage of labour

Second stage of labour

- Ensure fetal well-being
- Psychological support
- Analgesia

Admission to antenatal ward for support

Intrapartum care

Contractions stop

Contractions continue ± strengthen

Vaginal examination

<4 cm dilatation ± cervical effacement

>4 cm dilatation ± cervical effacement

Discharge home

Key learning points

Physiological considerations

Active and physiological management

Observations in the third stage

Management of retained placenta.

Introduction

The third stage of labour extends from the birth of the baby to the expulsion of the membranes and placenta.

The three commonest complications are:

- Delay in the third stage
- Retained placenta
- PPH (covered elsewhere).

The blood supply to the non-pregnant endometrium is a few mL per min, but, by the end of pregnancy, this figure has risen to 600–800 mL/min. Following delivery, this blood flow must be arrested promptly, and failure to do so will result in rapid and life-threatening blood loss. Indeed, on a global scale, death from PPH accounts for approximately 25% of all maternal deaths. Careful management of the third stage of labour is, therefore, essential to prevent serious maternal morbidity and mortality.

Physiology

Following separation of the placenta, bleeding from vessels in the placental bed is controlled by clotting of blood within uterine vessels supplying the placental bed. A number of physiological mechanisms come into operation, including:

- The powerful contraction and retraction of the uterus, especially the action of the interlacing of the myometrial fibres, sometimes known as 'living ligatures', which constrict the blood vessels running through the myometrium
- Pressure exerted on the placental site by the walls of the uterus, which contract firmly, with the walls in apposition, once the placenta and membranes have been delivered
- Blood clots in vessels in the placental bed.

The third stage of labour may be managed actively or physiologically.

Active management of the third stage

Active management of the third stage is routinely recommended, as it increases the duration of contraction, allowing the blood to clot; it reduces the risk of excess blood loss, following the birth, and can shorten the duration of the third stage.

The active management of the third stage involves a package of care which includes all of the following three components:

- Routine oxytocic use
- Early clamping and cutting of the cord
- Controlled cord traction (CCT).

The uterotonic of choice is oxytocin, 10 IU administered IM, with the birth of the anterior shoulder.

Physiological management of the third stage

Women at low risk of PPH who request physiological management of the third stage should be supported in their choice.

The physiological management of the third stage involves a package of care which includes all of the following three components:

- No routine oxytocic use
- No clamping of the cord until pulsation has ceased
- Delivery of the placenta by maternal effort.

Observations in the third stage of labour

Irrespective of the method of managing the third stage, observations by a midwife of a woman in the third stage include:

- Her general physical condition, as shown by her colour, respiration, and her own report of how she feels
- Vaginal blood loss
- Fundal height and uterine tone.

Delay in the third stage—retained placenta

NICE defines a third stage prolonged if not completed within 30 min of the birth of the baby with active management and within 60 min with physiological management.

The main risk is of haemorrhage, and this is more likely to occur following partial separation of the placenta or where it has separated completely but is retained within the uterus.

Initial steps

1. Ensure that oxytocin has been given and that the bladder is empty
2. Encourage skin-to-skin contact/breastfeeding
3. Ensure that the placenta is not simply retained within the vagina.

Management of retained placenta

1. Ensure IV access
2. Take blood for FBC and group and save (G & S)
3. Commence infusion of 30 U of Syntocinon® in 500 mL of 0.9% normal saline at 160 mL/h
4. Arrange for manual removal of placenta—this may be performed under regional anaesthesia. There is little evidence that umbilical vein injection of oxytocin reduces the need for manual removal.

Further reading

Cotter AM, Ness A, Tolosa JE (2001). Prophylactic oxytocin for the third stage of labour. *Cochrane Database of Systemic Reviews*, **4**, CD001808.

Nardin JM, Weeks A, Carroli G (2011). Umbilical vein injection for management of retained placenta. *Cochrane Database of Systemic Reviews*, **5**, CD001337.

National Institute for Health and Clinical Excellence (2007). *Intrapartum care: care of healthy women and their babies during childbirth*. NICE clinical guideline 55. Available at: <http://www.nice.org.uk/nicemedia/pdf/IPCNICEguidance.pdf>.

Algorithm for the management of the third stage of labour

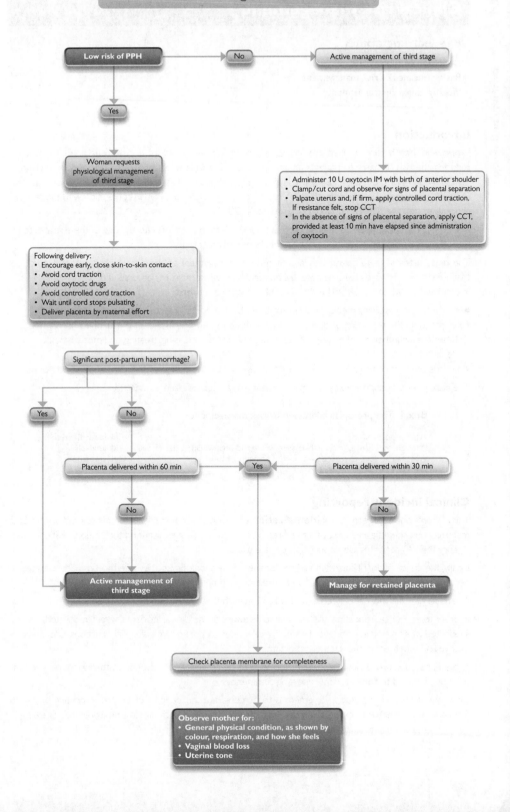

Clinical risk management

Key learning points

Definition of clinical risk
Basic principles of risk management
Investigating a clinical incident.

Introduction

Worldwide, health care systems are increasingly being obliged to adopt a systematic approach towards reducing the risk of harm to patients. Maternity care is particularly susceptible to risk, and, in England, in 2010/11, 8655 claims of clinical negligence against NHS bodies were received by the NHS Litigation Authority (NHSLA), up from 6652 claims in 2009/10. A total of £863 million was paid in connection with clinical negligence claims during 2010/11, up from £787 million in 2009/10.

The NHSLA has developed 50 risk management standards for maternity units, and one of these relates to the management of clinical incidents—as well as of claims and complaints.

The joint Australia/New Zealand standard defines risk management as 'the culture, processes and structures that are directed towards realizing potential opportunities whist managing adverse effects'.
In other words, when applied to health care, risk management is **not**:

- Primarily about avoiding medicolegal claims; it is instead a tool for improving the quality of care
- Simply about the reporting of clinical incidents—this is merely one aspect of the identification of risk. There are a number of other ways of identifying risk and for analysing, treating, and monitoring the identified risks
- Just the business of service managers—risk management is the business of all, clinicians and non-clinicians.

The basic principles addressed by risk management may be summarized, as in Box 1.

Box 1 The principles addressed by risk management

What could go wrong?	Risk **identification**
What are the chances of something going wrong and what would be the impact?	Risk **analysis**
What can be done to reduce the chance of something happening?	Risk **treatment**
What can we learn from what has gone wrong?	Risk **control**

Clinical incident reporting

This is simply one approach to risk **identification** by looking back at events when things went wrong. Each maternity unit should agree a list of agreed reporting incidents (trigger list), and the National Patient Safety Agency (NPSA) publishes lists of such appropriate triggers.

Ideally, the clinical incident forms should be completed electronically so they need to be made available on personal computers (PCs) in all clinical areas. Training in completing the forms is also essential.

The maternity unit must also agree a mechanism by which these forms can be processed.

In order to encourage reporting, all staff need to be aware of the clinical incident triggers, motivated, and feel supported when reporting incidents. Linking clinical incident reporting with disciplinary actions is counterproductive and simply encourages under-reporting.

A mechanism for processing the incident forms must be agreed, and personnel with responsibility for this must be identified **before** incident reporting commences.

One way of encouraging staff involvement is to demonstrate the benefits of incident reporting by regular feedback—a quarterly publication of 'incident reports that have led to a change in clinical practice', for example.

Although it is not the principal purpose of risk management in general, and incident reporting in particular, some adverse clinical incidents may lead to claims or complaints. If these are identified, then a process which handles them in a timely manner may mitigate subsequent damages. One such way in which this might happen is described in Key information.

Further reading

Department of Health (2000). *An Organisation with a memory: report of an expert advisory group on learning from adverse events in the NHS.* The Stationery Office, London.

Department of Health (2004). *Standards for better health.* Department of Health, London.

National Health Service Litigation Authority (2011). *Clinical negligence scheme for trusts. Maternity clinical risk management standards 2011/12.* NHLA, London. Available at: <http://www.nhsla.com>.

National Patient Safety Agency. Available at: <http://www.npsa.nhs.uk/>.

Royal College of Obstetricians and Gynaecologists (2009). *Improving patient safety: risk management for maternity and gynaecology.* Clinical governance advice No. 2. RCOG Press, London. Available at: <http://www.rcog.org.uk/files/rcog-corp/CGA2ImprovingPatientSafety2009.pdf>.

Key information for clinical risk management

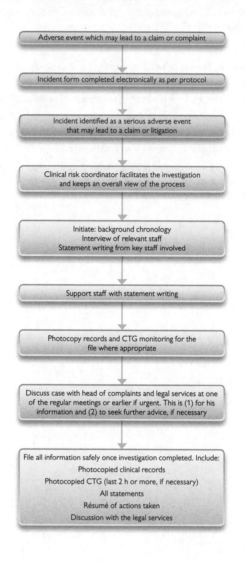

Adverse event which may lead to a claim or complaint

↓

Incident form completed electronically as per protocol

↓

Incident identified as a serious adverse event
that may lead to a claim or litigation

↓

Clinical risk coordinator facilitates the investigation
and keeps an overall view of the process

↓

Initiate: background chronology
Interview of relevant staff
Statement writing from key staff involved

↓

Support staff with statement writing

↓

Photocopy records and CTG monitoring for the
file where appropriate

↓

Discuss case with head of complaints and legal services at one
of the regular meetings or earlier if urgent. This is (1) for his
information and (2) to seek further advice, if necessary

↓

File all information safely once investigation completed. Include:
Photocopied clinical records
Photocopied CTG (last 2 h or more, if necessary)
All statements
Résumé of actions taken
Discussion with the legal services

Key information for clinical risk management

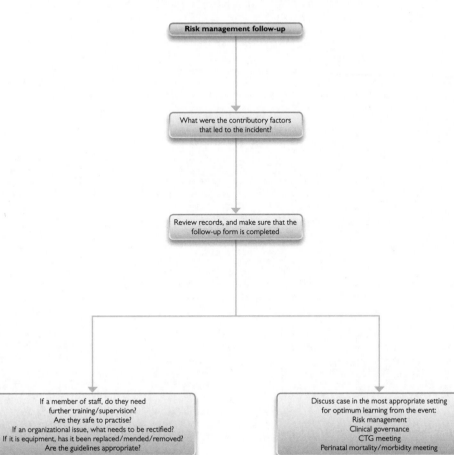

Risk management follow-up

What were the contributory factors that led to the incident?

Review records, and make sure that the follow-up form is completed

If a member of staff, do they need further training/supervision?
Are they safe to practise?
If an organizational issue, what needs to be rectified?
If it is equipment, has it been replaced/mended/removed?
Are the guidelines appropriate?

Discuss case in the most appropriate setting for optimum learning from the event:
Risk management
Clinical governance
CTG meeting
Perinatal mortality/morbidity meeting

SECTION 2

Obstetric emergency presentations

Vomiting in pregnancy

Key learning points
Hyperemesis occurs in 1–2% of pregnancies
Medical and surgical emergencies causing vomiting should be excluded
Early correction of dehydration and metabolic disturbance
Offer psychological support.

Introduction

Nausea and vomiting are often common features in early pregnancy, being experienced by up to 80% of pregnant women. It is thought to be due to physiological hormonal changes of the pregnant state. It often occurs around 8–10 weeks, although not exclusively confined to this period, and settles by 12–14 weeks. The symptoms are usually benign and short-lived.

The symptoms can be worse in multiple and molar pregnancy due to high circulating levels of serum β-hCG.

Hyperemesis gravidarum is defined as nausea and vomiting in pregnancy that is protracted and severe enough to cause electrolyte and metabolic derangements that can compromise maternal and fetal well-being. Hyperemesis can occur in about 1–2 % of all pregnancies. There is a high risk of recurrence in subsequent pregnancies.

Many medical and surgical emergencies can be associated with nausea and vomiting. Hence, it is important to identify the underlying cause and institute appropriate treatment.

Investigations

Should include:

- Urinalysis
  - MSU analysis for culture and sensitivity
- U + Es
- LFTs and thyroid function tests (TFTs)
- Pelvic USS for reassurance, to confirm viability, and to exclude molar and multiple pregnancy.

Exclude other causes

Infections: UTIs, including pyelonephritis; viral hepatitis; acute appendicitis; acute pancreatitis; CNS infections
Metabolic causes: diabetic ketoacidosis; hyperthyroidism
Gynaecological causes: torsion of ovarian cyst; red degeneration of fibroid.

Management principles

Immediate correction of dehydration, and electrolyte and metabolic disturbances
Antiemetics to stop further vomiting
Improve psychological well-being
Reassurance of the self-limiting nature of the condition
May require multidisciplinary approach to exclude other aetiology.

Thromboprophylaxis

Hyperemesis results in dehydration and is associated with bed rest, both of which are risk factors for thromboembolism. Thromboembolism deterrent (TED) stockings should be used, with a low threshold for giving prophylactic LMWH.

Antiemetics

These appear to be safe in the first trimester but are currently not licensed for use in pregnancy in the UK.

Vitamin supplementation

Should be given—especially thiamine to prevent Wernicke's encephalopathy in patients who have required IV fluids for >48 h or those with nutritional deficiency.

Pyridoxine (vitamin B1) may help to reduce severe nausea.

Antireflux measures

H2 receptor blockers (e.g. ranitidine) may be used in cases where dyspeptic symptoms accompany nausea and vomiting.

Severe refractory hyperemesis

Small studies have demonstrated a beneficial effect with the use of corticosteroids.
The regimen:

(a) Hydrocortisone, 100 mg IV tds, until vomiting controlled. If there is no response after 48 h, stop treatment

(b) If response is good, convert to oral prednisolone, 60 mg once daily. Then start decreasing the dose in 5 mg intervals every 2–3 days such that the patient is on the lowest dose of steroids which achieves adequate symptom control.

Enteral/parenteral nutrition

If the aforementioned measures are not successful, consider inserting a nasogastric tube (NGT) for feeding. Total parenteral nutrition (TPN) may become necessary in very severe cases of hyperemesis.

Further reading

Jewell D and Young G (2003). Interventions for nausea and vomiting in early pregnancy. *Cochrane Database of Systematic Reviews*, **4**, CD000145.

National Institute for Health and Clinical Excellence (2008). *Antenatal care: routine care of the healthy pregnant woman.* NICE clinical guideline 62. Available at: <http://www.nice.org.uk/nicemedia/pdf/cg062niceguideline.pdf>.

Nelson-Piercy C (2006). Gastrointestinal disease. In *Handbook of obstetric medicine*, 3rd edn, pp. 241–9. Informa Healthcare, London.

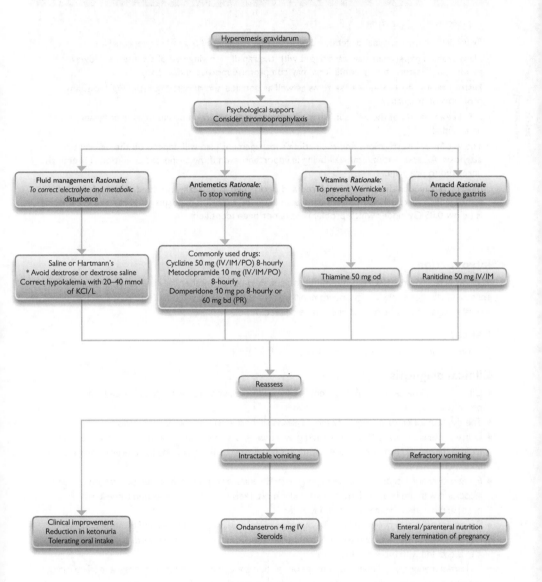

Abdominal pain in pregnancy

Key learning points

Resuscitation for maternal or fetal reasons must be considered urgently as appropriate

Many women experience pain associated with the rapidly growing size of the uterus. However, serious and life-threatening conditions may compromise mother and/or baby

History taking must include all systems as well as detailed and directed questioning about any problems of pregnancy

A full examination of the pelvis in early pregnancy or of the gravid uterus in later pregnancy must be included

The extent of investigations and the patient's management plan will depend on the differential diagnosis. Assessment of fetal well-being is important, even if the suspected condition is seemingly unrelated to pregnancy

Imaging techniques should be considered and performed as clinically indicated. Although fear of teratogenesis or childhood cancers causes anxiety, the radiation exposure of X-ray and CT imaging is below 0.05 Gy, under which problems have not been identified.

Introduction

Abdominal pain in pregnancy is a common problem. Pregnancy may alter the classical symptoms and signs of illness, and changes in physiology and immunity may influence investigation findings. As a result, achieving an accurate diagnosis may be difficult and can be delayed.

Causes

For complications relating to pregnancy, see Boxes 1, 2, and 3.

Clinical diagnosis

- Ultrasound is invaluable, helping to identify adnexal masses, intrauterine pregnancy, free fluid, or pelvic cysts
- The diagnosis of ectopic pregnancy should always be borne in mind and early gestation
- Urinary retention, owing to a retroverted gravid uterus, is an uncommon problem, usually occurring early in the second trimester. Catheterization is usually successful in allowing the uterus to rise into the abdomen
- Functional ovarian cysts are normal in pregnancy. Bleeding or rupture may occur, but torsion is usually associated with the heavier dermoid cyst and is more likely to occur in the second trimester or in post-partum when the uterus rapidly involutes
- Round ligament pain occurs in 10–30% of pregnancies, usually in the mid-second trimester, and is characterized by pain situated towards the uterine fundus and laterally downwards to the groin. The pain is exacerbated with movement and walking
- UTIs, pyelonephritis, and maternal renal pelvis dilation are common problems in pregnancy. The clinical presentation is often clear, as the pain and tenderness are classically from loin to groin
- Renal and ureteric colic are uncommon, owing to the physiological ureteric dilatation occurring in pregnancy

> **Box 1** Early pregnancy
>
> Miscarriage
> Ectopic pregnancy
> Ruptured/bleeding corpus luteum
> Acute urinary retention (retroverted uterus)
> Round ligament strain

Box 2 Later pregnancy

Labour
Abruption
Braxton–Hicks
Chorioamnionitis
Uterine rupture or scar dehiscence
Acute fatty liver
Pre-eclampsia/HELLP syndrome
Fibroid degeneration
Round ligament strain
SPD

Box 3 Causes of abdominal pain unrelated to pregnancy

Include all medical and surgical problems, including:
Urinary tract—infection, pyelonephritis, renal pelvis dilatation, hydronephrosis, stones
GI—appendicitis, dyspepsia, cholecystitis, pancreatitis, gastritis, perforation
Vascular disorders—sickle cell disease, ruptured aneurysm, thrombosis
Rare causes—trauma, pneumonia, porphyria

- Abruption is a potentially life-threatening event for mother and baby. A rapid decision may be necessary to establish whether delivery is necessary and by what means
- Uterine scar dehiscence is more common, usually occurs in labour and following induction. Fetal compromise may precede the overt signs and symptoms of pain, peritonism, change of abdominal/uterine contour, and shock
- The diagnosis of appendicitis (1 in 2000 pregnancies) may be difficult in pregnancy. The appendix, behind the gravid uterus, is pushed upwards towards the right upper quadrant of the abdomen. Signs of peritonitis may be less marked, the expected neutrophilia less pronounced and may not be significantly elevated above pregnancy levels
- SPD (1 in 36 to 1 in 300) pain and instability can be severe and are usually associated with movement and particularly hip abduction
- Spontaneous intra-abdominal bleeding is rare, but 25% of splenic artery ruptures occur in pregnancy.

Further reading

American College of Obstetricians and Gynecologists (1995). *Guidelines for diagnostic imaging during pregnancy. ACOG Committee Opinion No. 158.* ACOG, Washington, DC.

Algorithm for abdominal pain in pregnancy

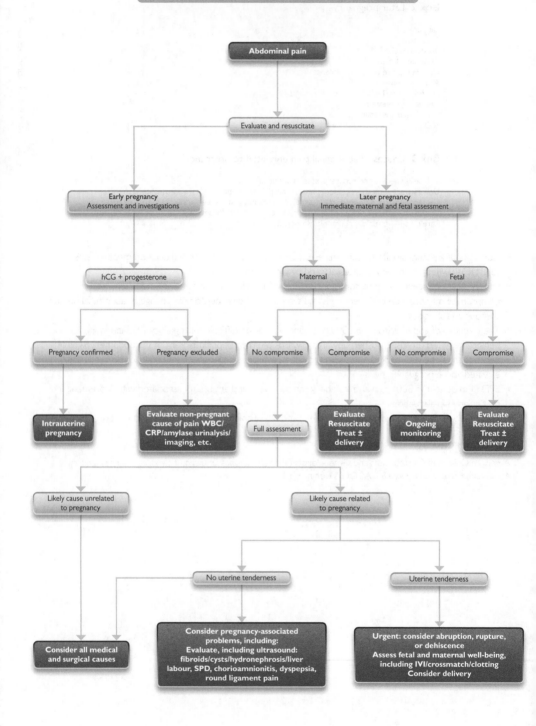

Bleeding in late pregnancy (antepartum haemorrhage)

Key learning points

Potential for life-threatening bleeding

Early resuscitation and identification of cause

Senior involvement

Balance of risks to mother vs risk of prematurity.

Introduction

Antepartum haemorrhage (APH) complicates 3–5% of pregnancies and is defined as bleeding from or into the genital tract, occurring from 24 + 0 weeks of pregnancy and prior to the birth of the baby. The amount of bleeding can vary from 'spotting' to profuse haemorrhage, leading to significant maternal or fetal mortality or morbidity.

The most important causes of APH are placenta praevia and placental abruption, although these are not the most common.

Placenta praevia

The placenta is located over, or is in close proximity to, the internal cervical os. Incidence is about 1 in 250 pregnancies.

The placenta normally implants in the upper segment. In about 5% of cases, the placenta covers the internal os at mid-pregnancy. In the majority of cases, because of subsequent development of the lower uterine segment, the placenta appears to 'migrate' away from the os.

- Grade 1: placenta in the lower segment but does not reach the internal os
- Grade 2: lower edge of placenta reaches, but does not cover, the internal os
- Grade 3: placenta partially covers the internal os
- Grade 4: placenta completely covers the entire internal cervical os.

Placenta accreta

A morbidly adherent placenta, associated with a high maternal morbidity and mortality. The risk is higher in an anterior, low-lying placenta and a previous uterine scar.

Placenta accreta typically presents as painless vaginal bleeding.

Diagnosis is by ultrasound examination. Transvaginal ultrasound scan (TVS) is safe and more accurate than abdominal scan.

Antenatal inpatient vs outpatient management

Women with placenta praevia in the third trimester should be counselled that the bleeding tends to be recurrent, with increasing severity with subsequent bleeds, and their care should be tailored to their individual needs.

Mode of delivery

If the placental edge is <2 cm from the internal os in the third trimester, delivery is likely to be by C/S. This carries a risk of massive obstetric haemorrhage and may result in hysterectomy. Hence, delivery should be carried out in a unit with a blood bank and high dependency care facilities, with a consultant obstetrician and consultant anaesthetist in attendance.

Placental abruption

Defined as premature separation of a normally sited placenta. Bleeding is usually sudden and is associated with severe, continuous pain. Bleeding can be revealed (65–80%) when it escapes into the vagina or concealed (20–35%) when it accumulates behind the placenta with no external evidence of bleeding.

The amount of revealed bleeding has poor correlation with the severity of abruption. DIC occurs in about 10% of abruptions, due to the release of thromboplastin into the maternal circulation with placental separation, and is more common with fetal death.

Risk factors

- Pre-eclampsia
- Multiple pregnancy
- Polyhydramnios
- Previous history of abruption
- Cocaine use
- Trauma (accidental/domestic violence)
- Smoking.

As the clinical presentation is variable, management should be guided by the severity of the abruption and maternal and fetal condition. Delay can be fatal to the fetus.

Further reading

Royal College of Obstetricians and Gynaecologists (2011). *Antepartum haemorrhage*. Green-top guideline No. 63. Available at: <http://www.rcog.org.uk/files/rcog-corp/GTG63_05122011APH.pdf>.

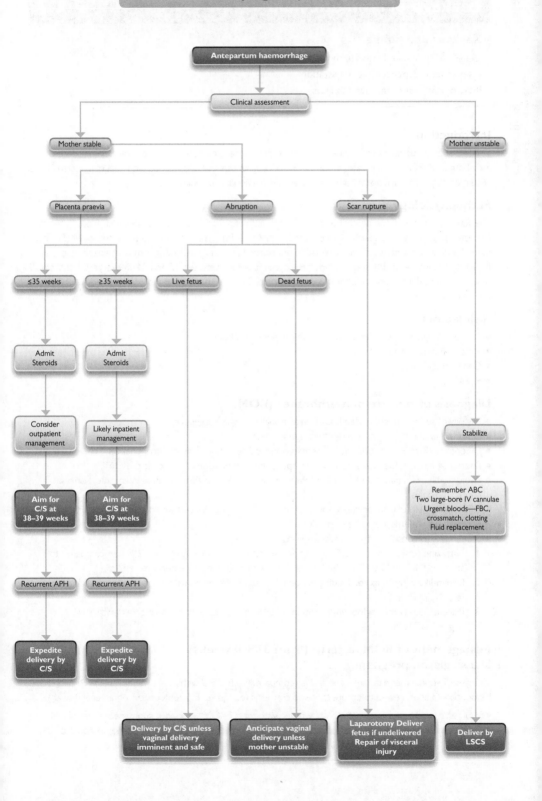

Algorithm for bleeding in late pregnancy

Antepartum haemorrhage

Clinical assessment

Mother stable

Mother unstable

Placenta praevia

Abruption

Scar rupture

≤35 weeks

≥35 weeks

Live fetus

Dead fetus

Admit Steroids

Admit Steroids

Consider outpatient management

Likely inpatient management

Stabilize

Aim for C/S at 38–39 weeks

Aim for C/S at 38–39 weeks

Remember ABC
Two large-bore IV cannulae
Urgent bloods—FBC, crossmatch, clotting
Fluid replacement

Recurrent APH

Recurrent APH

Expedite delivery by C/S

Expedite delivery by C/S

Delivery by C/S unless vaginal delivery imminent and safe

Anticipate vaginal delivery unless mother unstable

Laparotomy Deliver fetus if undelivered Repair of visceral injury

Deliver by LSCS

Leakage of amniotic fluid

Key learning points
Identification of membrane rupture
Risks to fetus dependent upon gestation
Risks of infection to mother and fetus.

Introduction
Leakage of amniotic fluid occurs when the amniotic membrane ruptures. Preterm prelabour rupture of the membranes (PPROM) complicates around 2–3% of pregnancies and is associated with 40% of preterm births. Fetal mortality is through prematurity, sepsis, and/or pulmonary hypoplasia.

Pathophysiology
The fetus is contained in a protective bag with the amniotic fluid that also provides a cushion. In the first trimester, production of amniotic fluid is from the placenta, but, from the second trimester, it switches over to fetal production, with a constant circulation of urination and fetal swallowing. Amniotic fluid is essential for fetal lung maturity. A critical stage of lung development occurs between 16 and 24 weeks' gestational age. If there is minimal fluid or anhydramnios occurs prior to 20 weeks, then pulmonary hypoplasia develops, which can be lethal.

Risk factors
- Previous pregnancy complicated by PPROM or preterm labour
- Antepartum bleeding
- Genital tract infection
- Smoking.

Diagnosis of rupture of membranes (ROM)
- History of sudden, uncontrolled loss of fluid vaginally is highly suggestive
- History may also be vague with slight leakage/wetness
- Differential diagnoses include vaginal discharge and leakage of urine/stress incontinence
- Pooling of liquor in the posterior fornix on **speculum examination** is diagnostic of ROM
- Avoid digital examination, unless absolutely necessary, because of the risk of ascending infection and chorioamnionitis
- USS may be helpful in inconclusive speculum examinations—a reduced amniotic fluid index with a normally grown fetus would be suggestive
- Other tests to consider if the diagnosis is in doubt include:
  1. **Nitrazine** (testing pH of the fluid)—vaginal secretions are acidic (pH 3.8–4.2) when compared to amniotic fluid (pH 7.0–7.3). This test has high rates of false positive/negative results.
  2. **Insulin-like growth factor binding protein 1**—can be measured with point-of-care dipstick test (e.g. Actim Prom®)
  3. **Placental alpha microglobulin-1 protein**—can be measured with point-of-care device (e.g. AmniSure®).

Management of ROM at term (from 37 + 0 weeks) in a singleton pregnancy
The risk of serious neonatal infection is 1% (compared with 0.5% with intact membranes). The antenatal history should be reviewed to ensure there no concerns (e.g. group B Streptococcus on antenatal swab).

- Women should be advised that 60% of women with term PROM will labour spontaneously within 24 h
- Consideration should be given to induction of labour to prevent neonatal infection if not in labour by 24 h

- If expectant management beyond 24 h is chosen by the woman:
    1. Low vaginal swabs and C-reactive protein (CRP) should not be performed unless clinically indicated
    2. Women should be advised to record temperature every 4 h during waking hours and to report immediately any change in colour/smell of their vaginal loss
    3. Women should be informed that bathing/showering is not associated with an increased risk in infection, but sexual intercourse might be
    4. Fetal movements and FHR should be assessed every 24 h.

Management of ROM at 34 + 0 to 36 + 6 weeks in singleton pregnancy with no complications

Management is controversial. Evidence available is unclear on whether prolongation of pregnancy to 37 + 0 or to deliver from 34 + 0 weeks is better for neonatal outcome. Randomized controlled trials (e.g. PPROMT) are ongoing to answer this question.

Management of ROM at 23 + 0 to 33 + 6 weeks

(See also Chapter 38 on preterm labour.) Conservative management is indicated, unless there are additional obstetric indications (e.g. infection or fetal compromise).

- The aim is to reach greater maturity without intervening chorioamnionitis developing
- Close maternal and fetal monitoring is warranted
- Perform low vaginal swab, FBC, and CRP to exclude infection
- Assess maternal pulse, temperature, respiratory rate, and BP
- Note colour of liquor and uterine tenderness
- Admit to hospital for initial observation, if there are suspicions of infection, or for antibiotic treatment
- Provided no evidence of sepsis or preterm labour are present, it is common UK practice to discharge the woman home, with close surveillance as an outpatient through a maternity day assessment unit
- Outpatient management should include observation of the woman for clinical symptoms and signs of infection, including self-measurement of temperature (± pulse) every 4–8 h
- Weekly vaginal swab, FBC, and CRP—these tests have poor sensitivities, with significant false positives.

Interventions for PPROM

1. Antenatal glucocorticosteroids—should be given and reduce the risk of respiratory distress syndrome (RDS), intraventricular haemorrhage (IVH), and necrotizing enterocolitis (NEC) in the infant

2. Antibiotic prophylaxis—is associated with a significant reduction in chorioamnionitis (RR 0.66, 95% CI 0.46–0.96), neonatal infection (RR 0.67, 95% CI 0.52–0.85), use of surfactant (RR 0.83, 95% CI 0.72–0.96), oxygen therapy (RR 0.88, 95% CI 0.81–0.96), and abnormal cerebral USS prior to discharge (RR 0.81, 95% CI 0.68–0.98) and delays delivery. Oral erythromycin 250 mg four times daily for 10 days should be given

3. Tocolysis—is controversial, with little proven benefit in improving perinatal mortality or morbidity.

At present, there are insufficient data to support the use of supplementary progesterone, tissue sealants, or amnioinfusion.

Further reading

National Institute for Health and Clinical Excellence (2007). *Intrapartum care: care of healthy women and their babies during childbirth*. NICE clinical guideline 55. Available at: <http://www.nice.org.uk/nicemedia/live/11837/36275/36275.pdf>.

National Institute for Health and Clinical Excellence (2008). *Induction of labour*. NICE clinical guideline 70. Available at: <http://www.nice.org.uk/nicemedia/live/12012/41255/41255.pdf>.

Royal College of Obstetricians and Gynaecologists (2006). *Preterm prelabour rupture of membranes*. Green-top guideline No. 44. Available at: <http://www.rcog.org.uk/files/rcog-corp/GTG44PPROM28022011.pdf>.

Algorithm for leakage of amniotic fluid

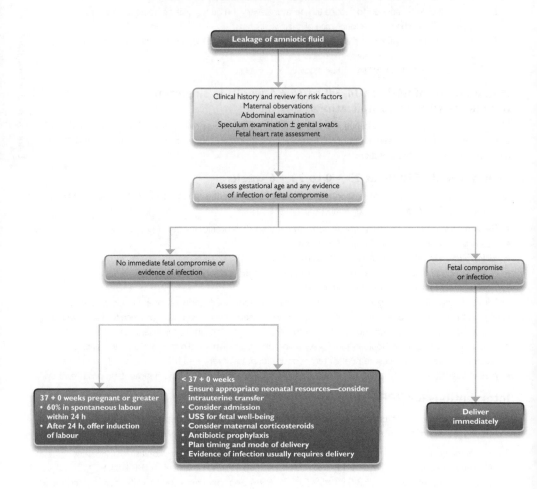

Convulsions

Key learning points

Convulsions carry significant risk to mother and fetus

A fit in pregnancy should be treated as eclampsia unless proven otherwise

Appropriate neuroimaging essential if no clear cause identified.

Causes

- Obstetrically related (eclampsia)
- Prior CNS disease (epilepsy)
- Electrolyte imbalance
- Metabolic problem
- Hypoxia
- Space-occupying lesion
- Endocrinopathy
- Drug use
- Trauma
- Infection
- Vascular accident.

All patients who present with their first seizure in pregnancy, other than eclampsia, should have imaging of the brain with CT or MRI and be reviewed by a neurologist. Most women with epilepsy have been diagnosed before conception.

Epilepsy

In women with known seizure disorder, pre-pregnancy counselling is important to discuss the control of seizures, advisability of getting pregnant, and the risks involved. If the woman has been seizure-free for >2 years, consideration should be given to stopping the drugs. Opportunity should be taken to find out whether the fits are well controlled and review/substitute the dosages and medications that are relatively contraindicated in pregnancy, e.g. sodium valproate, as well as to advise taking prophylactic folic acid to reduce the incidence of birth defects. The risk of the fetus developing epilepsy subsequently is about 4% if one parent is affected and up to 15% if both parents are affected.

Effect of pregnancy on seizure control is unpredictable. Most patients show no change in seizure frequency during pregnancy. However, patients with frequent seizures (>1 per month) often deteriorate during pregnancy. This may be due to the lowered serum levels of anticonvulsants, secondary to increased blood volume. There is also an accelerated metabolism of anticonvulsants during pregnancy. Patients on anticonvulsants may develop folate deficiency and megaloblastic anaemia. They may also develop a deficiency of vitamin K-dependent procoagulants, which may lead to an increased risk of bleeding at delivery.

Women on anticonvulsants have an increased risk of fetal congenital malformations (5–10%). The most common abnormalities are craniofacial defects and NTDs. It must be remembered that the drug-related teratogenic risk to the fetus is less than the risk to the fetus from maternal epileptic seizures. There is a slightly increased risk of haemorrhagic disease in the fetus due to depletion of vitamin K-dependent coagulation factors and increased risk of fetal demise with status epilepticus.

Monotherapy with the lowest required dose is always preferred during pregnancy (carbamazepine is commonly used). Dividing doses and reducing peak blood levels of drugs are beneficial. Medication should not be altered in pregnancy if well controlled, and compliance should be emphasized. Alpha-fetoprotein, fetal anomaly screening in early pregnancy, and vitamin K supplementation at term are important. If seizure control becomes difficult, it should be made sure that the patient is taking her anticonvulsants regularly; obtain a serum level of the drug, and consult a neurologist. An increase in drug dosage may be required. In such cases, the dose will have to be reduced in the first week following delivery to avoid toxic effects. The patient should return to her neurologist for subsequent management and follow-up in the non-pregnant state.

Seizure in pregnancy

If an episode of convulsion occurs during pregnancy, it is important to find out if the seizure was observed, as a description is useful for diagnosis, concentrating on where it started, how it progressed, and whether it was localized or generalized. The associated mental status, presence of antecedent vomiting, headache, fever, visual changes, and post-ictal confusion or paralysis are also helpful. Physical examination should be thorough, with special attention to neurologic and ocular findings.

Eclampsia

Consider any pregnant woman who has generalized convulsions to have eclampsia until proven otherwise. Characteristic signs of pre-eclampsia, such as hypertension, proteinuria, and hyperreflexia, make eclampsia the most likely diagnosis. Progressive hyperreflexia with clonus generally precedes the seizures. The diagnosis may be complicated if severe hypertension produces a secondary intracranial haemorrhage. Laboratory studies should include a baseline FBC, platelet count, U + Es, LFTs, uric acid, blood sugar, and urine analysis. Electroencephalography may be needed to diagnose epilepsy. A CT scan/MRI of the brain and a cerebral angiogram may also be required to make a definite diagnosis of an intrinsic CNS disorder such as an aneurysm, arteriovenous malformation, neoplasm, thromboembolism, or bleeding.

Management of eclamptic seizure

- Follow the 'ABC' approach, with protection of airway as a priority
- Magnesium sulfate and antihypertensives should be administered to prevent further seizures or hypertensive complications
- When stable, efforts should be made to deliver the fetus. In the presence of a mature fetus, unless vaginal delivery is imminent, serious consideration should be given to Caesarean delivery
- Fluid and electrolyte imbalance should be corrected. Appropriate medications should be administered, using diazepam or phenytoin, which adequately control seizures without compromising the vital functions.

Mode of delivery

Vaginal delivery should be the aim in non-eclamptic causes. Vitamin K is given to the mother from 37 weeks to prevent bleeding complications post-delivery due to clotting factor deficiency. C/S is indicated only for obstetrical reasons or for status epilepticus. Vaginal delivery is preferable, except in cases of increased intracranial pressure in which labour may be contraindicated. The second stage may be shortened with assisted instrumental delivery. After delivery, the baby should be given vitamin K, and breastfeeding is not contraindicated.

Further reading

Nelson-Piercy C (2010). Neurological problems. In *Handbook of obstetric medicine*, 4th edn, pp. 151–75. Informa Healthcare, London.

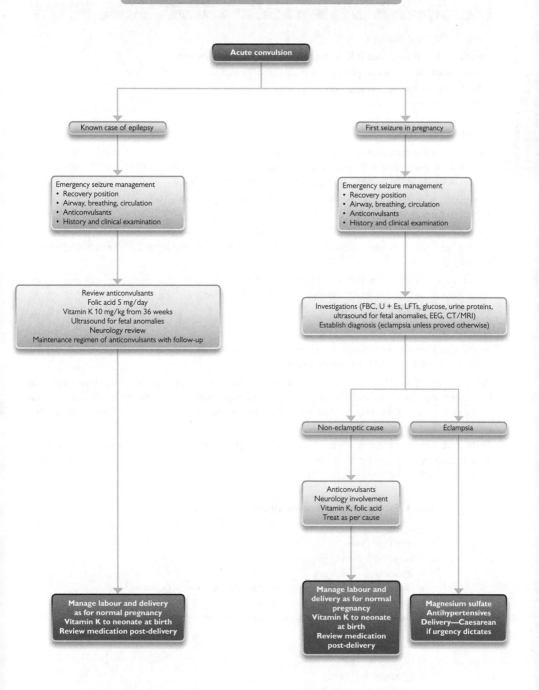

Algorithm for acute convulsion

Acute convulsion

Known case of epilepsy

Emergency seizure management
• Recovery position
• Airway, breathing, circulation
• Anticonvulsants
• History and clinical examination

Review anticonvulsants
Folic acid 5 mg/day
Vitamin K 10 mg/kg from 36 weeks
Ultrasound for fetal anomalies
Neurology review
Maintenance regimen of anticonvulsants with follow-up

Manage labour and delivery as for normal pregnancy
Vitamin K to neonate at birth
Review medication post-delivery

First seizure in pregnancy

Emergency seizure management
• Recovery position
• Airway, breathing, circulation
• Anticonvulsants
• History and clinical examination

Investigations (FBC, U + Es, LFTs, glucose, urine proteins, ultrasound for fetal anomalies, EEG, CT/MRI)
Establish diagnosis (eclampsia unless proved otherwise)

Non-eclamptic cause

Anticonvulsants
Neurology involvement
Vitamin K, folic acid
Treat as per cause

Manage labour and delivery as for normal pregnancy
Vitamin K to neonate at birth
Review medication post-delivery

Eclampsia

Magnesium sulfate
Antihypertensives
Delivery—Caesarean if urgency dictates

Reduced fetal movements

Key learning points

Reduced fetal movements (RFMs) may imply poor placental function

Women should be encouraged to report significant reduction in fetal movement

RFM warrants further investigation.

Fetal movements

Fetal movements are considered a sign of well-being.

Perception of fetal movements ranges widely. There is no accepted definition of RFM. It is the mother's perception of decreased movements over 24 h that is of clinical importance.

Primigravid women usually perceive fetal movements (quickening) by 20–22 weeks' gestation and by 16–18 weeks in subsequent pregnancies.

A regular pattern of fetal movements has diurnal variation—with increased movements in the afternoon and evening. Fetal movements are usually absent during spells of fetal sleep, lasting for 20–40 min throughout the day and night.

During poor placental function and hypoxia, the fetus may respond by reducing fetal movements. An absence or decrease in fetal movements should be considered a warning sign, being associated with an increased risk of stillbirth.

Background

Five to 15% of women report RFM during pregnancy. However, 70% of those with a single episode of RFM and no other risk factors have a normal outcome.

Women tend to perceive most movement when lying down and resting. If a woman is unsure about fetal movements after 28 weeks' gestation, it is recommended that she lies on her left side and focusses on fetal movements for 2 h. If she does not feel ten or more movements within these 2 h, she should contact her midwife or maternity unit.

There is **no** benefit in adopting any specific formal 'kick count' alarm limit. It is recommended that women should recognize their baby's individual patterns of movements, and, if they are concerned about RFM, they should contact their midwife.

Box 1 Factors affecting fetal movements

- Maternal
  - Maternal activity
  - Increased maternal weight
  - Smoking
  - Drugs, e.g. alcohol, benzodiazepines, barbiturates, narcotics, methadone
  - Corticosteroids for fetal lung maturation
  - Maternal illness, e.g. anaemia, hypothyroidism, metabolic disorders
- Fetal/intrauterine
  - Fetal sleep
  - Intrauterine death
  - Placental insufficiency
  - Fetal anaemia or hydrops
  - Anterior placenta
  - Polyhydramnios
  - Congenital fetal abnormality (neurological/skeletal).

There are also a number of factors (see Box 1) that limit the perception, or actual number, of fetal movements.

It has been shown that between 11 and 29% of women presenting with RFM carry an SGA fetus (less than the 10th centile), with approximately 5% having severe growth restriction.

Management of RFM

On first presentation

Less than 28 weeks' gestation:
  Fetal heartbeat should be confirmed by Doppler auscultation
  Assess for risk factors
  In the presence of risk factors or a suspicion of poor fetal growth, an ultrasound assessment should be considered

After 28 weeks' gestation:
  Immediate reassurance of FHR activity
  Distinguish between those pregnancies with fetal compromise and/or at future risk (see Box 2)
  In the absence of any risk factors, the woman should be reassured and no additional vigilance is required
  Women should be encouraged to report any further RFM so that additional evaluation may be undertaken.

Clinical examination should include maternal pulse rate, BP, temperature, urine analysis, and the assessment of the abdomen and uterine size (measurement of the symphysis fundal height (SFH) in cm.

CTG should be performed for at least 20 min to exclude fetal compromise.

If there are any additional risk factors for fetal growth restriction or stillbirth, even in the place of a normal CTG, an **USS** should be performed, preferably within 24 h of presentation.

Ultrasound **assessment of liquor volume** should be undertaken to assess amniotic fluid index (AFI). If AFI is <5 cm, this is associated with poor outcome.

Ultrasound **fetal biometry**, including an abdominal circumference measurement, is indicated in cases where SFH measurement suggests an SGA fetus or in the place of oligohydramnios. A review of fetal morphology may be offered.

Management of recurrent RFMs

There is an increased risk of poor perinatal outcome associated with further or recurrent episodes of RFM. Ultrasound should be performed, and continuing monitoring of the pregnancy or IOL should be considered by a senior clinician.

Box 2 Risk factors linked with stillbirth and poor obstetric outcome

- Recurrent RFM
- Known fetal growth restriction
- Maternal hypertension/pre-eclampsia
- Diabetes
- Poor obstetric history (previous stillbirth or growth restriction)
- Extremes of maternal age
- Primiparity
- Smoking, obesity
- Placental insufficiency
- Fetal congenital malformation
- Racial/ethnic factors.

Conclusion

A reduction in fetal movements is common in pregnancy. A perception of RFM leads to maternal anxiety that may be compounded by unnecessary investigation of, or intervention in, otherwise uncomplicated pregnancies. However, RFM may indicate a fetus at risk, and full assessment is mandatory.

Further reading

Royal College of Obstetricians and Gynaecologists (2011). *Reduced fetal movements*. Green-top guideline No. 57. Available at: <http://www.rcog.org.uk/files/rcog-corp/GTG57RFM25022011.pdf>.

Unterscheider J, Horgan R, O'Donoghue K, Greene R (2009). Reduced fetal movements. *The Obstetrician & Gynaecologist*, **11**, 245–53.

Algorithm for reduced fetal movements

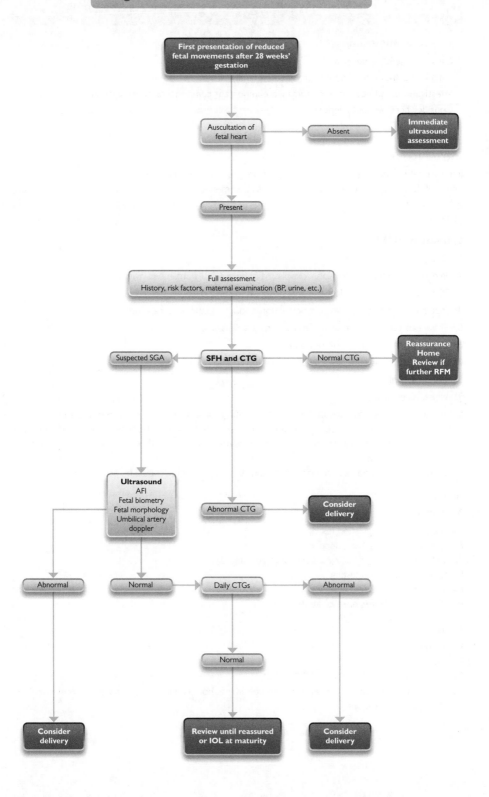

Intrauterine death

Key learning points

Cause frequently unknown

Timing of delivery should take into account family wishes

Investigations and post-natal debriefing are important components of management

Consider bereavement support.

Introduction

Intrauterine fetal death (IUFD) at any stage of pregnancy is extremely distressing for the parents. The incidence of IUFD is about 6 per 1000 total births in women aged 20–34 years but tends to be higher at the extremes of reproductive life. By definition, stillbirth is any fetus born with no signs of life after 24 weeks of gestation.

Causes of IUFD

1. Congenital malformations
2. Infections—Listeria, Chlamydia, Toxoplasma, rubella, CMV, human parvovirus
3. Maternal lupus anticoagulant and antiphospholipid antibodies
4. Maternal disorders—diabetes, hypertension, endocrinopathy, trauma, uterine rupture
5. FMH—abruption, vasa praevia, fetomaternal transfusion
6. Isoimmunization—either Rh or non-Rh
7. Uteroplacental insufficiency—IUGR, prolonged pregnancy
8. Cord accidents
9. Unexplained factors.

In the absence of obvious precipitating event, the diagnosis is often first suspected due to RFM. Further suspicion is raised when the fetal heart cannot be auscultated, and the diagnosis is confirmed by USS. The diagnosis should be revealed to the parents in a sensitive way, allowing them adequate privacy and time to deal with the bad news.

If the cause is not obvious, a thorough history and clinical examination should be performed.

Investigations

Maternal

Haematology and coagulation testing

Biochemistry, including liver function

Thrombophilia screen, including antiphospholipid antibodies

Infection and serological testing

Blood group and antibody screening

Parental karyotyping (where indicated).

Fetal

Karyotype

Fetal swabs

Placental pathology

Post-mortem examination—if parents decline, consider a more restricted post-mortem, biopsies, and/or radiological investigations.

Management of IUFD

Although the onset of spontaneous labour may be awaited following IUFD, in the majority of cases, labour will need to be induced due to maternal request or to prevent the risks of infection and coagulopathy. Recommendations about labour and birth should take into account the mother's preferences as well as her medical condition and previous intrapartum history.

Women should be strongly advised to take immediate steps towards delivery if there is sepsis, pre-eclampsia, placental abruption, or membrane rupture, but a more flexible approach can be discussed if these factors are not present.

Well women, with intact membranes and no laboratory evidence of coagulopathy, should be advised that they are unlikely to come to physical harm if they delay labour for a short period.

Women who delay labour for periods longer than 48 h should be advised to have testing for coagulopathy twice weekly. There is a 10% chance of maternal DIC within 4 weeks from the date of fetal death and an increasing chance thereafter.

If a woman returns home before labour, she should be given a 24-h contact number for information and support. Women contemplating prolonged expectant management should be advised that the value of post-mortem may be reduced. Vaginal birth is the recommended mode of delivery for most women, but Caesarean birth will need to be considered with some.

Method of induction of labour

Mifepristone (200 mg) should be used 48 h prior to the administration of prostaglandins for cervical ripening. Oral misoprostol should be used in a dosage of 100 micrograms 6-hourly before 26 weeks, and 25–50 micrograms 4-hourly at 27 weeks or more. Appropriate analgesia (diamorphine) should be offered, and experienced supportive midwifery care is vital. In general, ARM should be delayed as long as reasonably possible, as the risk of chorioamnionitis is increased in comparison to the live birth.

Antibiotics may be needed if there is evidence of infection, and cabergoline is the drug of choice for suppression of lactation.

After delivery, the parents should be offered an opportunity to see or hold the baby if they desire and be given photographs or hand/foot prints of the baby if they wish. Bereavement counselling and support should be organized for the parents before discharge from the delivery suite. A named midwife for easy contact with a telephone number and a definitive date for follow-up to review the results and plan the care for future pregnancies should be arranged.

Timely completion of stillbirth registration documents is vital to assist the family during this tragic time.

Further reading

Royal College of Obstetricians and Gynaecologists (2010). *Late intrauterine fetal death and stillbirth*. Green-top guideline No. 55. Available at: <http://www.rcog.org.uk/files/rcog-corp/GTG%2055%20Late%20Intrauterine%20fetal%20death%20and%20stillbirth%2010%2011%2010.pdf>.

Care pathway for intrauterine death

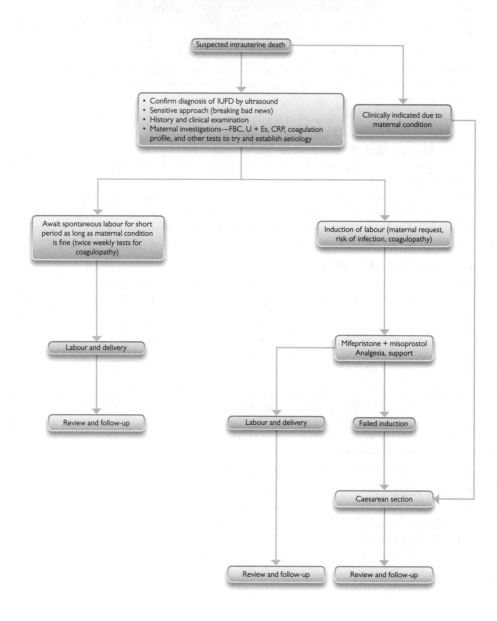

Breech presentation

Key learning points

Breech presentation complicates 3–4% of singleton term pregnancies

External cephalic version has a success rate of 40–50%

For the term breech, C/S is the safest mode of delivery, but vaginal breech delivery may be reasonable in selected cases

The safest mode of delivery for the preterm breech is unclear.

Introduction

Often, there are no definite causative factors for breech presentation at term, but polyhydramnios, uterine abnormality, placenta praevia, or cornual implantation are associated factors.

Types of breech

The denominating joints are the fetal knees when referring to flexion and extension.

1. Extended breech (frank breech): the knees are extended, and the hips are flexed. The fetus has its feet near its ears—a position which can persist briefly after birth. Accounts for 60–70% of all cases

2. Flexed breech (complete breech): the knees and hips are flexed, creating a more irregular presenting part. There is a slightly higher incidence of cord prolapse. The least common type accounting for 10% of breeches

3. Footling or kneeling breech (incomplete breech): one or both feet, or knees may present. The small diameter of these parts may deliver through an incompletely dilated cervix, resulting in entrapment of the fetal head.

Risks

- Increased mortality and morbidity, compared with vertex
- More susceptible to hypoxia and trauma; C/S is not always protective, particularly in the case of rough handling of preterm breeches at C/S.

Management

External cephalic version (ECV)

Converting breech presentation into vertex is a well-described procedure. An attempt is made by manipulating the fetus abdominally to move the fetus from a breech to a vertex presentation.

- ECV should be done at around 36–37 weeks, in order to minimize the risk of reversion to breech
- Overall success rate is around 50%
- Tocolysis increases the success rate
- Complications are rare and include loss of variability on the CTG or fetal bradycardia; very rarely, uterine rupture
- ECV should only be conducted in a setting where facilities exist for emergency C/S
- Contraindications to ECV are where Caesarean delivery is required, APH within the last 7 days, abnormal CTG, major uterine anomaly, ruptured membranes, and multiple pregnancy (except delivery of second twin).

Management of delivery

Caesarean section vs vaginal breech delivery

The Term Breech Trial is still the most important evidence driving the practice of breech delivery. C/S carries the risk of major surgery for the mother but, at term, is the safest mode of delivery for the fetus. There are no long-term follow-up studies.

Assisted vaginal breech delivery

If considering planned vaginal breech delivery, the following should be considered as adverse factors:

- Other contraindications to vaginal birth (e.g. placenta praevia, compromised fetal condition)
- Clinically inadequate pelvis
- Footling or kneeling breech presentation
- Large baby (usually defined as larger than 3800 g)
- Growth-restricted baby (usually defined as smaller than 2000 g)
- Hyperextended fetal neck in labour (diagnosed with ultrasound or X-ray where ultrasound is not available)
- Lack of presence of a clinician trained in vaginal breech delivery
- Previous C/S.

Undiagnosed breech in the second stage of labour provides a difficult clinical challenge. Second-stage C/S carries a higher maternal and fetal morbidity and is not guaranteed to be protective against fetal injury.

- An epidural anaesthetic is useful but not essential
- Continuous fetal heart monitoring is essential
- Buttock fetal blood sampling (FBS) is not recommended
- Role of augmentation with synthetic oxytocin is controversial
- Accurate diagnosis of full dilatation of the cervix is essential, as a foot or knee may prolapse through a partially dilated cervix, leading the clinician to prematurely undertake manoeuvres which result in entrapment of the fetal head in the cervix
- Breech extraction should not be performed routinely
- The following three principles should guide decision making during delivery:
  1. Do not hurry
  2. Do not apply traction—'hands off the breech'
  3. Maintain a sacro-anterior position
- Having achieved satisfactory progress to full dilatation and carefully confirmed there is no cervix felt, allow the buttocks to deliver spontaneously. Consider an episiotomy at this point. Allow descent to occur between each manoeuvre. Deliver extended legs by gentle flexion at the knee joint. Allow further descent. The arms may deliver spontaneously; alternatively, this can be assisted at this juncture by sweeping them across the chest with a finger in the antecubital fossa. Applying traction before delivery of the arms will cause them to be raised above the fetal head (nuchal arm), causing difficulty in delivering the aftercoming head—this can be overcome by rotating the shoulders towards the fingers of the displaced arm. Once the scapulae are visible, use Lovset's manoeuvre to deliver the shoulders (femoropelvic grip and rotation through 180°), then deliver the arm as described
- The fetal head may deliver spontaneously
- There are three ways to achieve controlled delivery of the aftercoming head:
  1. Forceps to the aftercoming head (Pipers or alternative low or mid-cavity forceps)
  2. Mauriceau–Smellie–Viet manoeuvre
  3. Burns–Marshall manoeuvre—note concerns about hyperextension of fetal neck.

Further reading

Hannah EM, Hannah WJ, Hewson SA, et al. (2000). Planned caesarean section versus planned vaginal birth for breech presentation at term: a randomised multicentre trial. *Lancet*, **356**, 1375–83.

Royal College of Obstetricians and Gynaecologists (2006). *External cephalic version and reducing the incidence of breech presentation*. Guideline No. 20a. Available at: <http://www.rcog.org.uk/files/rcog-corp/uploaded-files/GT20aExternalCephalicVersion.pdf>.

Royal College of Obstetricians and Gynaecologists (2006). *The management of breech presentation*. Guideline No. 20b. Available at: <http://www.rcog.org.uk/files/rcog-corp/GtG%20no%2020b%20Breech%20presentation.pdf>.

Society of Obstetricians and Gynaecologists of Canada (2009). *Vaginal delivery of breech presentation*. Clinical guideline No. 226. Available at: <http://www.sogc.org/guidelines/documents/gui226CPG0906.pdf>.

Algorithm for breech presentation

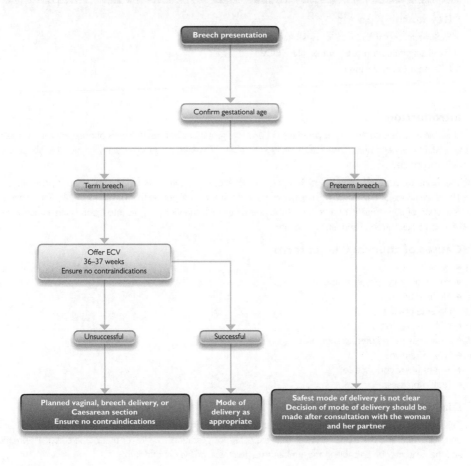

Unstable lie

Key learning points

Exclude maternal and fetal causes once diagnosis made

Stabilizing induction is an option after ECV

C/S requires senior input.

Introduction

Unstable fetal lie is commonly encountered at preterm gestations before 36 weeks of pregnancy. If it persists as unstable or becomes transverse or oblique lie after 37 weeks, it can significantly impact the labour and delivery process.

The incidence is approximately 1 in 300 pregnancies and may result in shoulder, limb, or cord presentation. There are no major hazards to the fetus or mother in the antenatal period from an abnormal lie. Spontaneous resolution of abnormal lie occurs in 85% of cases by term. If the woman goes into labour with an abnormal lie, it increases maternal and fetal morbidity.

Causes of abnormal lie at term

- Wrong dates
- Prematurity and preterm labour
- Multiparity
- Placenta praevia
- Multiple pregnancy
- Pelvic masses and uterine anomalies
- Polyhydramnios
- Severe pelvic contracture
- Fetal anomalies.

Diagnosis

This is based on history (to confirm dating) and clinical examination. The maternal abdomen often appears unusually wide, and the fundus is lower than expected for gestation. The lower uterine pole appears empty, and the head may be palpable in the lumbar area, iliac fossa, or hypochondrium.

Pelvic examination (contraindicated if placenta praevia is suspected) reveals an empty pelvis, or a prolapsed limb/cord or shoulder that may be felt through the cervix. Once an abnormal lie is diagnosed, an attempt should be made to establish the possible cause. Ultrasound examination should be performed to confirm fetal lie and placental localization and to try to identify any obvious cause.

Management

When transverse or oblique lie is diagnosed at or before 36 weeks, and provided placenta praevia, fetal anomalies, uterine anomalies, multiple pregnancy, and fetal compromise are ruled out, ECV may, in some cases, be attempted. If this is successful and the fetus remains stable as a cephalic presentation, the rest of the antenatal care can be normal. If ECV fails or there is persistent unstable lie, there is a risk of prolapsed umbilical cord or obstructed labour if the woman enters labour or has SROM with abnormal lie. In these cases, it is best to admit the woman to the antenatal ward so that, at the earliest signs of labour, ECV can be performed or immediate C/S be carried out, should there be SROM and prolapse of the cord or arm.

If the fetus stabilizes to cephalic presentation spontaneously or after ECV at 38 weeks or more, a stabilizing induction can be performed. This includes admission to the labour ward; the lie is corrected to longitudinal lie with a vertex presentation, if necessary, followed by oxytocin infusion, as per the normal induction protocol. Once contractions have established and the cervix is favourable, a pelvic examination is performed and amniotomy carried out with abdominal hand holding the head in the pelvis after excluding cord presentation.

In all other cases of transverse lie or after unsuccessful ECV, elective C/S is recommended at 39 weeks or beyond. Caesarean for transverse lie requires the presence of an experienced obstetrician and crossmatched blood. On occasions, delivery can prove difficult, and acute tocolysis or vertical uterine incision may become necessary for safe delivery of the baby.

Abnormal lie in established labour is managed by emergency C/S.

Further reading

Mackenzie IZ (2010). Unstable lie, malpresentations, and malpositions. In D James, P Steer, C Weiner, B Gonik, eds. *High risk pregnancy: management options*, 4th edn, pp. 1123–38. Elsevier Saunders, St Louis.

Algorithm for unstable lie

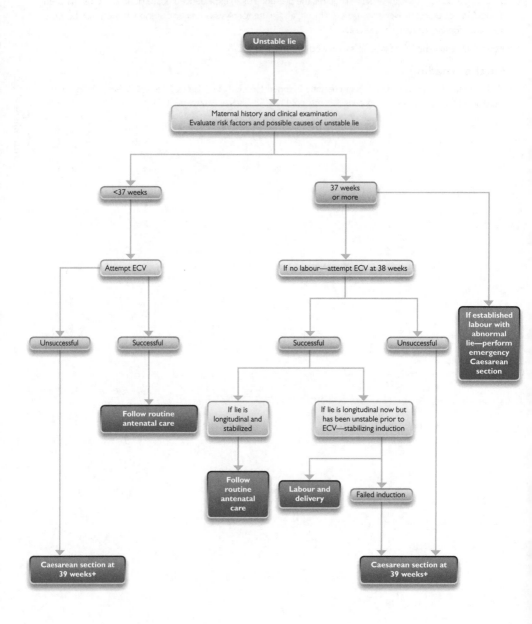

Preterm labour (PTL)

Key learning points

Aetiology largely unknown

Neonatal prognosis dependent on gestation at delivery

Give antenatal steroids once diagnosis confirmed

Tocolysis indicated to achieve delay to allow steroid administration and *in utero* transfer.

Introduction

Preterm birth is defined as birth <37 + 0 weeks of gestation. Five to 9% of births in Europe are preterm. Fetal viability in the UK is defined as from 24 + 0 weeks, although, increasingly, 'rescue' of fetuses from 23 + 0 weeks is being attempted.

- 5% of preterm births occur at <28 weeks (extreme prematurity)
- 15% at 28–31 weeks (severe prematurity)
- 20% at 32–33 weeks (moderate prematurity)
- 60–70% at 34–36 weeks (late preterm).

The underlying mechanism of PTL is poorly understood and probably multifactorial.

Neonatal prognosis

Complications include:

- Death
- Neurodevelopmental handicap
- Cerebral palsy
- RDS
- NEC.

When counselling prospective parents:

- Use figures/proportions of survival for the neonates of **women in labour**
- Figures of survival to discharge of those neonates who enter the neonatal intensive care unit can be falsely reassuring of high survival.

EPICure 2 data for extreme prematurity are presented in Table 1.

Risk factors

- Previous history
- Multiple pregnancy—60% of twins deliver by 36 weeks
- Polyhydramnios
- Previous cervical surgery
- PPROM
- Race—black women have twice the risk (15–18%)
- Extremes of reproductive age (<18 years or >35 years).

Principles of management

Review medical history and details of this and previous pregnancies for risk factors:

1. Symptoms
   - Abdominal pains—contraction-type pains of increasing severity
   - Vaginal bleeding—abruption may precipitate labour
   - ROM
   - Associated symptoms, e.g. UTI

Table 1 Survival and disability—an alternative approach to expressing the figures from EPICure 2—of 100 babies delivered at 23, 24, or 25 weeks' gestation, what happens to them? (figures in brackets are actual numbers in the EPICure 2 cohort)

Gestation in weeks	23	24	25
Alive at onset of labour/prior to C/S	100 (416)	100 (494)	100 (550)
Number alive at birth	81 (339)	89 (442)	95 (521)
Died on delivery suite	29 (122)	12 (61)	4 (23)
Admitted to NICU	52 (217)	77 (381)	91 (498)
Died on NICU	36 (151)	41 (203)	27 (152)
Discharged home	*16 (66)*	*36 (178)*	*63 (346)*
Survival without major morbidity: defined as any of severe abnormality on cerebral USS, severe BPD, retinopathy of prematurity stage ≥3 or laparotomy for NEC	*4 (15)*	*11 (52)*	*24 (133)*
At 30 months old			
Severe disability	4 (17)	7 (37)	10 (57)
Moderate disability	3 (14)	7 (33)	9 (48)
No disability	8 (32)	22 (107)	43 (236)

*BPD, bronchopulmonary dysplasia; NEC, necrotizing enterocolitis; NICU, neonatal intensive care unit. Denominator is number alive at onset of labour. Data from Kate L Costeloe, Enid M Hennessy, Sadia Haider, Fiona Stacey, Neil Marlow, Elizabeth S Draper. Short term outcomes after extreme preterm birth in England: comparison of two birth cohorts in 1995 and 2006 (the EPICure studies). BMJ 2012;**345**:e7976; and Tamanna Moore, Enid M Hennessy, Jonathan Myles, Samantha J Johnson, Elizabeth S Draper, Kate L Costeloe, Neil Marlow. Neurological and developmental outcome in extremely preterm children born in England in 1995 and 2006: the EPICure studies. BMJ 2012;**345**:e7961.*

2. Signs
   - Abdominal palpation—contractions, presentation
   - Speculum examination—look for ROM, bleeding, whether cervix is open, cervical length. Obtain high vaginal swab (HVS)
   - Vaginal examination—if speculum uninformative
3. Assess fetal well-being
   - CTG—individual units will decide criteria for gestational age when CTG will influence management
   - Consider transabdominal ultrasound—assess fetal biometry with estimated fetal weight (EFW), umbilical artery Doppler, and amniotic fluid assessment. For significant prematurity (23–32 + 0 weeks), EFW can be used alongside gestational age to predict survival
4. Basic investigations
   - FBC and CRP to exclude infection
   - Urinalysis and exclude UTI
5. Transvaginal (TV) scan for cervical length and/or assessment of fetal fibronectin may be useful.

Differential diagnosis

Pregnancy-specific:

- Abruption, Braxton–Hicks pains, round ligament pain.

Other condition:

- UTI, pyelonephritis, appendicitis, cholecystitis.

Management

1. Ensure adequate local neonatal facilities—consider whether safe to transfer *in utero* to unit with appropriate facilities

2. Antenatal corticosteroids to mother—reduction in RDS with use of either betamethasone or dexamethasone IM injections. Aim to give 24–48 h prior to delivery. Duration of effect is around 7 days. Concerns with regard to neurodevelopmental effects on infant with repeated courses

3. Tocolysis—limited evidence that tocolysis improves perinatal mortality or morbidity; mainly used to facilitate *in utero* transfer or to prolong pregnancy to allow timely steroid administration. Main drugs used are calcium antagonists (nifedipine) or oxytocin receptor blocker (atosiban).

4. Magnesium sulfate—IV infusion, 4 g loading dose, followed by 1 g/h infusion. Reduces risk of cerebral palsy by 50%. Consider use in imminent preterm delivery, e.g. cervical dilation ≥4 cm with regular contractions. Exact gestational age to use is debatable—Australian guidance suggests use in PTL <30 weeks

5. Fetal monitoring strategy—for extreme prematurity (23 + 0 to 26 + 0 weeks), sensitive discussion required with patient and family about monitoring strategy and actions to take if fetal concerns. Options include no monitoring, intermittent auscultation, or continuous CTG. Make parents aware that, if they opt for CTG interpretation, it is frequently difficult and recommended delivery interventions, such as C/S, may risk maternal health. Most UK units adopt the use of CTG monitoring at 26 + 1 weeks

6. Mode of delivery—individualize, depending on clinical circumstances. Many will deliver rapidly and vaginally. C/S for preterm breech has not been shown to be protective. If C/S is necessary for extreme prematurity, classical C/S may be needed

7. **Therapeutic interventions not been shown to improve outcome**
   1. Antibiotics—data from Oracle study do not support use of routine antibiotics in PTL with intact membranes
   2. Progestogens—may have role in prevention (particularly in asymptomatic women with short cervix on TV scan of 10–20 mm) but, in symptomatic PTL, not proven to improve outcome.

Further reading

Costeloe KL, Hennessy EM, Haider S, Stacey D, Marlow N, Draper ES (2012). Short term outcomes after extreme preterm birth in England: comparison of two birth cohorts in 1995 and 2006 (the EPICure studies). *BMJ*, **345**, e7976.

Moore T, Hennessy EM, Myles J, *et al.* (2012). Neurological and developmental outcome in extremely preterm children born in England in 1995 and 2006: the EPICure studies. *BMJ*, **345**, e7961.

Royal College of Obstetricians and Gynaecologists (2010). *Antenatal corticosteroids to reduce neonatal morbidity and mortality.* Green-top guidance No. 7. Available at: <http://www.rcog.org.uk/womens-health/clinical-guidance/antenatal-corticosteroids-prevent-respiratory-distress-syndrome-gree>.

Royal College of Obstetricians and Gynaecologists (2011). *Tocolysis for women in preterm labour.* Green-top guidance No. 1b. Available at: <http://www.rcog.org.uk/womens-health/clinical-guidance/tocolytic-drugs-women-preterm-labour-green-top-1b>.

Royal College of Obstetricians and Gynaecologists (2011). *Magnesium sulphate to prevent cerebral palsy following preterm birth.* Scientific Advisory Committee Opinion Paper 29. Available at: <http://www.rcog.org.uk/files/rcog-corp/28.9.11SACMagnesium.pdf>.

Care pathway for preterm labour

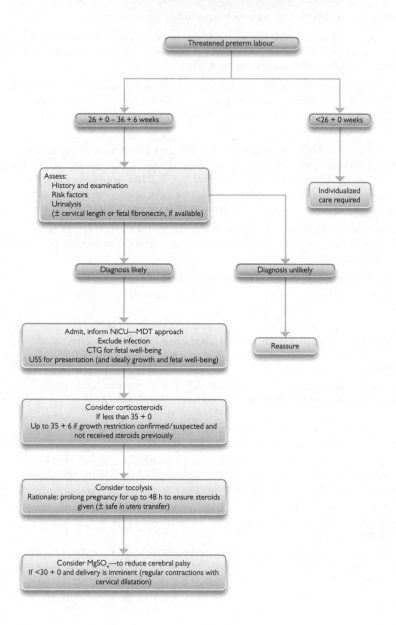

Threatened preterm labour

26 + 0 – 36 + 6 weeks

<26 + 0 weeks

Assess:
  History and examination
  Risk factors
  Urinalysis
  (± cervical length or fetal fibronectin, if available)

Individualized care required

Diagnosis likely

Diagnosis unlikely

Admit, inform NICU—MDT approach
Exclude infection
CTG for fetal well-being
USS for presentation (and ideally growth and fetal well-being)

Reassure

Consider corticosteroids
If less than 35 + 0
Up to 35 + 6 if growth restriction confirmed/suspected and not received steroids previously

Consider tocolysis
Rationale: prolong pregnancy for up to 48 h to ensure steroids given (± safe *in utero* transfer)

Consider MgSO$_4$—to reduce cerebral palsy
If <30 + 0 and delivery is imminent (regular contractions with cervical dilatation)

Poor progress in labour

Key learning points

Multifactorial nature of poor progress in labour requires detailed assessment

The partogram is an essential adjunct for the identification and management of poor progress

Augmentation in multiparous women should be performed with great care.

Poor progress in labour is associated with increased maternal morbidity and mortality. Prolonged labour can predispose to maternal dehydration, sepsis, and ketoacidosis and increase the risk of PPH, obstetric fistulae, obstruction, uterine rupture, stillbirth, and maternal death. There is also an increase in C/S rates for dystocia and failure to progress, with its attendant risks for both the mother and the baby. Systematic evidence-based management of poor progress in labour can prevent adverse obstetric outcomes.

Latent phase of labour

Slow progress in the latent phase should be managed conservatively. With a reactive CTG trace and absence of any maternal medical or obstetric complications, the woman may be reassured and offered analgesia and ambulation until active phase is established.

First stage of labour

Delayed progress of labour in the active first stage is diagnosed when the rate of cervical dilatation falls below 0.5 cm/h. On the partogram, this may be identified when the progress line falls to the right of the alert line, drawn at 1 cm/h in the active phase of labour. Action must be taken if there has been <2 cm progress in cervical dilatation over 4 h.

The three Ps should be remembered while looking for the cause of poor progress:

Power of uterine contractions

Passenger, i.e. fetal size or position

Passage (or **P**elvis).

Primary dysfunctional labour

Diagnosed when the progress of labour is slow, right from the beginning of the active first stage, usually due to inefficient uterine activity.

Secondary arrest

Diagnosed when the rate of progress slows after initial adequate cervical dilatation, commonly malposition or cephalopelvic disproportion, with or without efficient uterine activity.

Assessments

Assessments should include:

- Review of maternal history and risk factors
- Abdominal palpation to feel for frequency and duration of contractions and fetal size
- CTG
- Colour of liquor
- Maternal hydration
- Pain relief
- Vaginal examination (4-hourly) to assess presentation, position, station, synclitism, caput, and moulding.

Management

Slow progress in the first stage should be managed actively, with regular maternal and fetal assessments, use of partogram, ARM, prompt administration of oxytocin when indicated, pain relief, adequate hydration, and close support for the woman and partner from medical staff.

ARM should be followed by reassessment in 2 h and oxytocin augmentation added, if required, especially in nulliparous women. When labour is augmented in parous women, they must be closely monitored due to increased risks of hyperstimulation and uterine rupture.

Generally, an 8-h period of augmentation of labour, in the absence of signs of cephalopelvic disproportion, will result in the majority of women progressing to a vaginal delivery. However, if labour fails to progress, despite adequate augmentation, or there are added complications (such as pathological CTG, disproportion suggested by increasing caput, and moulding with no, or minimal, descent or malpresentation), then a C/S is indicated.

Further reading

National Institute for Health and Clinical Excellence (2007). *Intrapartum care: management and delivery of care to women in labour.* NICE clinical guideline 55. Available at: <http://guidance.nice.org.uk/CG55>.

Algorithms for poor progress in labour

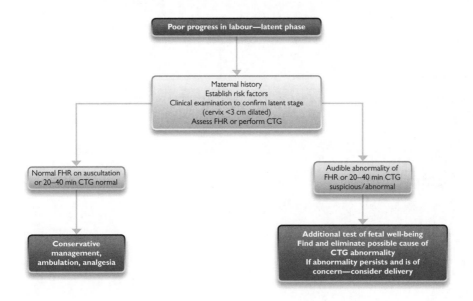

Algorithms for poor progress in labour

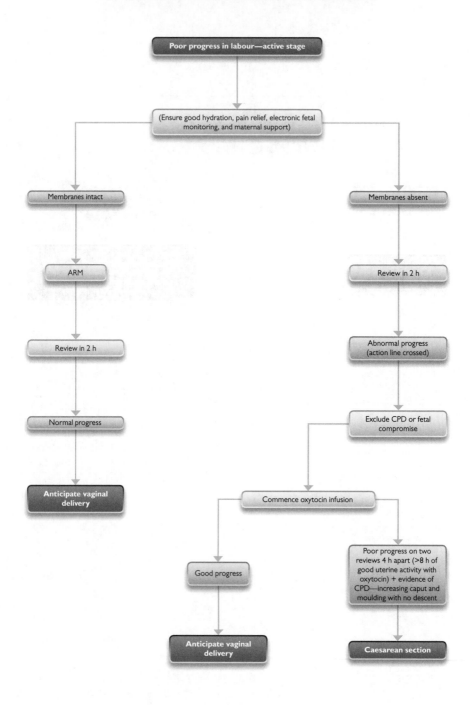

Abnormal fetal heart rate in labour

Key learning points

Analysis of the CTG can give an indication of fetal well-being

Classification of heart rate abnormalities allows detailed planning and prioritization of subsequent management.

Introduction

Appropriate management of abnormal fetal heart rate (FHR) patterns in labour is critical to ensure fetal well-being and avoid adverse obstetric outcomes. Action required depends upon the stage of labour, nature of abnormality of the trace, and the fetal reserve. Fetuses with low reserve tend to become hypoxic more rapidly in the presence of heart rate abnormalities.

Indicators of potential low reserve

- Post-term
- IUGR
- Intrapartum bleeding
- Moderate to thick meconium, with scanty amniotic fluid
- Intrauterine infection
- Prematurity.

Interpretation of the CTG

The presence of accelerations, normal baseline heart rate (110–160 bpm), variability of more than 5 bpm, and absence of any decelerations are features of a normal reassuring CTG. With a normal baseline CTG, a gradually developing hypoxia will be reflected by no accelerations, repeated decelerations that tend to get deeper and wider, and gradually rising baseline rate. On the other hand, if the baseline CTG is non-reactive with reduced baseline variability, the development of further abnormal features with progress of labour are variable and subtle. These may be difficult to recognize, because there might be pre-existing hypoxia and the fetus is unable to respond.

UK guidelines promote a systematic approach to CTG interpretation, with individual features classified as reassuring, non-reassuring, or abnormal, and the overall CTG as normal/suspicious/pathological (see Tables 1 and 2). Continuous EFM should be systematically assessed at least once an hour in active labour and more often if indicated. Abnormal CTG features include:

- Baseline tachycardia
- Reduced baseline variability (<5 bpm)
- Repeated atypical variable
- Repeated late decelerations
- A prolonged deceleration (>3 min)
- A sinusoidal pattern to the heart.

Table 1 Classification of FHR trace features

Feature	Baseline (bpm)	Variability (bpm)	Decelerations	Accelerations
Reassuring	110–160	≥5	None	Present
Non-reassuring	100–109 161–180	<5 for 40–90 min	Typical variable decelerations, with >50% of contractions occurring for over 90 min Single prolonged deceleration for up to 3 min	The absence of accelerations with otherwise normal trace is of uncertain significance
Abnormal	<100 >180 Sinusoidal pattern ≥10 min	< 5 for 90 min	Either atypical variable decelerations, with >50% of contractions, or late decelerations, or both for over 30 min Single prolonged deceleration for >3 min	

Table 2 Definition of normal, suspicious, and pathological FHR traces (NICE)

Category	Definition
Normal	FHR trace in which all four features are classified as reassuring
Suspicious	FHR trace with one feature classified as non-reassuring and the remaining features classified as reassuring
Pathological	FHR trace with two or more features classified as non-reassuring or one or more classified as abnormal

These features warrant action, depending on the stage of labour and classification of the severity of the CTG abnormality. It must always be remembered that, with any given CTG trace, the clinical actions and decisions will vary, depending on the overall clinical picture.

Management of the suspicious and pathological CTG

Generally, a 'suspicious' CTG can be managed conservatively. A 'pathological' CTG requires scalp FBS where appropriate/feasible; otherwise, delivery should be expedited.

Suspicious CTG

Interventions for a suspicious trace will depend on the suspected underlying cause of the abnormal FHR. Simple measures include:

- Changing maternal position
- Treating hypotension
- Treating pyrexia
- Rehydration
- Reducing or stopping oxytocin
- Tocolysis for hyperstimulation.

Pathological CTG

Scalp FBS for pH analysis and lactate measurement is recommended with pathological CTGs to identify those fetuses that require delivery. In the absence of facilities to perform FBS, acceleration of the FHR to fetal acoustic stimulation or with vaginal examination is reassuring. An abnormal FBS (pH ≤7.20) result indicates immediate delivery of the fetus. If the FBS result is normal (pH ≥7.25), sampling should be repeated no more than 1 h later if the FHR trace remains pathological or sooner if there are further abnormalities. After a borderline FBS result (pH 7.21–7.24), sampling should be repeated no more than 30 min later if the FHR trace remains pathological or sooner if there are further abnormalities. The time taken to obtain FBS needs to be considered when planning repeat samples. If the FHR trace remains unchanged and the FBS result is stable after the second test, a third/further sample may be deferred, unless additional abnormalities develop on the trace. Where a third FBS is considered necessary, senior obstetric opinion should be sought and the overall clinical picture reviewed to consider whether delivery is indicated.

Timing is crucial in cases of prolonged decelerations of <80 bpm for longer than 3 min, and urgent intervention is required. Possible causes of prolonged decelerations include abruption, cord prolapse, and scar rupture.

In the event of a catastrophic event, such as bradycardia, immediate delivery should be considered, and the '3, 6, 9, 12, 15 minute' guidance can be followed. Interventions, such as cessation of oxytocin and treatment of maternal hypotension, should commence immediately. If there are no signs of recovery at 6 min, preparations should be made to transfer to theatre by 9 min. C/S should commence by 12 min, with the aim of delivery by 15 min. If instrumental delivery is possible, this should be achieved within 15–20 min; a difficult instrumental delivery should, however, be avoided. An experienced neonatal team should attend the delivery if resuscitation is anticipated.

A large number of cases will recover by 9 min, and C/S may not be necessary, unless there are additional reasons for concern. Appropriate debriefing and explanation of events to the mother and partner should follow.

Further reading

National Institute for Health and Clinical Excellence (2007). *Intrapartum care: management and delivery of care to women in labour.* NICE clinical guideline 55. Available at: <http://guidance.nice.org.uk/CG55>.

Algorithm for abnormal fetal heart rate in labour

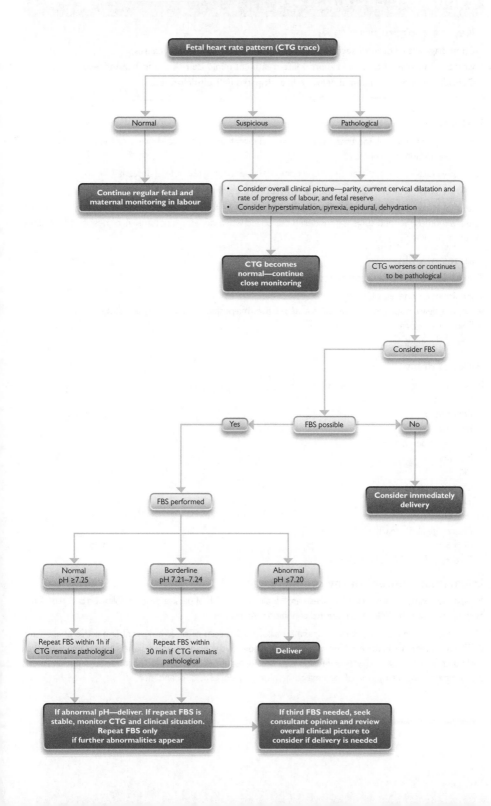

Prolonged second stage

Key learning points

Upon diagnosis of delayed second stage, assess for maternal and fetal causes

Correct diagnosis of cause and appropriate treatment minimize risk to mother and fetus

Consider 'trial of instrumental delivery' in anticipated difficult deliveries.

Definition

Second stage of labour is the time from full cervical dilatation (10 cm) to delivery of the fetus. The second stage is divided into two phases:

1. 'Passive phase'—where uterine contractions continue to bring about fetal descent
2. 'Active phase'—once maternal bearing down efforts begin.

Birth should take place within 3 h of the start of second stage for nulliparous women and within 2 h for multiparous women. Second stage is considered prolonged when delivery is not imminent despite 1 h of active maternal pushing.

Causes of delay

The main causes for delayed second stage are:

- Inefficient uterine activity
- Cephalopelvic disproportion which may be relative (malposition of the head) or absolute
- Epidural analgesia
- Maternal exhaustion.

Risks of delay

Maternal
   Exhaustion
   Dehydration
   Ketoacidosis
   Operative delivery
   Infection
   PPH
   Uterine rupture
Fetal
   Infection
   Heart rate abnormalities
   Hypoxia
   Trauma from a difficult delivery.

Usual management of the second stage

Nulliparous women with epidural analgesia are usually allowed 2 h of passive descent, followed by 1 h of active pushing, as long as the fetal and maternal condition remains well.

Multiparous women with epidural analgesia are allowed 1 h each of passive descent and active phase if the CTG remains normal. In the extra hour which is allowed with the epidural analgesia, it is important to maintain good uterine activity, and oxytocin infusion may be started if needed. Delayed second stage in multiparous women must raise a suspicion of fetal malposition or cephalopelvic disproportion.

Management of prolonged second stage

Once prolonged second stage is diagnosed, the obstetrician should review the clinical findings and consider instrumental delivery or C/S.

Assessment should include:

- Maternal condition (pulse, BP, temperature, ketonuria)
- Fetal condition (CTG and presence of meconium)
- Abdominal examination to determine the size of baby and descent of the head
- Vaginal examination to note station of head, synclitism, degree of caput, moulding, and position of the vertex
- Uterine contractions should be at a frequency of 4–5 every 10 min, each lasting >45 s
- Maternal hydration status.

Judicious use of oxytocin (after ruling out disproportion or fetal compromise) should be ensured. Blood should be crossmatched and an IV line established if assisted delivery is contemplated. In the presence of FHR abnormalities, if assisted delivery cannot be safely accomplished, C/S should be considered.

In most cases, it will be clear that the head is in low or outlet position and that assisted delivery will be accomplished with ease. However, in those cases in which the fetal head is arrested in between spines to +1 station, it is often prudent to declare 'a trial of instrumental delivery'. If difficulties are encountered during such delivery, the obstetrician can immediately abandon the procedure and proceed to C/S. This takes away the pressure from the obstetrician to persist with an attempt at vaginal delivery and minimizes risks to both the mother and fetus.

A difficult second-stage delivery may be associated with PPH from uterine atony and/or trauma and shoulder dystocia. These should be anticipated and appropriately managed.

Further reading

National Institute for Health and Clinical Excellence (2007). *Intrapartum care: management and delivery of care to women in labour.* NICE clinical guideline 55. Available at: <http://guidance.nice.org.uk/CG55>.

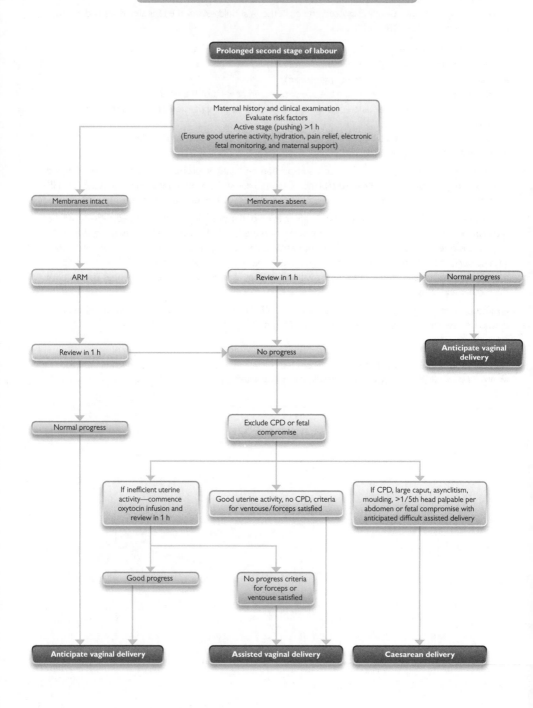

Algorithm for prolonged second stage of labour

Prolonged second stage of labour

Maternal history and clinical examination
Evaluate risk factors
Active stage (pushing) >1 h
(Ensure good uterine activity, hydration, pain relief, electronic fetal monitoring, and maternal support)

Membranes intact

Membranes absent

ARM

Review in 1 h

Normal progress

Review in 1 h

No progress

Anticipate vaginal delivery

Normal progress

Exclude CPD or fetal compromise

If inefficient uterine activity—commence oxytocin infusion and review in 1 h

Good uterine activity, no CPD, criteria for ventouse/forceps satisfied

If CPD, large caput, asynclitism, moulding, >1/5th head palpable per abdomen or fetal compromise with anticipated difficult assisted delivery

Good progress

No progress criteria for forceps or ventouse satisfied

Anticipate vaginal delivery

Assisted vaginal delivery

Caesarean delivery

Post-partum haemorrhage (PPH)

Key learning points

PPH remains a major cause of morbidity and mortality

The amount of blood lost is frequently underestimated

Rapid instigation of well-rehearsed protocols for the management of PPH saves lives.

Definition

The traditional definition of primary PPH is the loss of 500 mL or more of blood from the genital tract within 24 h of delivery of a baby. Secondary PPH is defined as abnormal or excessive bleeding from the genital tract between 24 h and 6 weeks post-natally. PPH can be minor (500–1000 mL), major (>1000 mL), or massive (loss of 30–40% of maternal blood volume, with moderate to severe circulatory compromise).

Epidemiology

PPH is one of the leading causes of maternal death worldwide; it occurs in about 10.5% of births and accounts for over 130 000 maternal deaths annually.

Causes

- Uterine atony
  - Accounts for about 70% of cases
  - Risk factors include placenta praevia, multiple pregnancy, previous PPH, Asian ethnicity, obesity (BMI >35), prolonged labour (>12 h), big baby (>4 kg), and nulliparous women over the age of 40
- Trauma
  - Accounts for about 20% of cases
  - Risk factors include delivery by C/S, operative vaginal delivery, episiotomy, and big baby (>4 kg)
- Retained tissue
  - Accounts for about 10% of cases and is due to retention of placental tissue
- Coagulopathy
  - Accounts for about 1% of cases
  - Risk factors include placental abruption, pre-eclampsia, pyrexia in labour, and major PPH.

Prevention

Most cases of PPH have no identifiable risk factors. Active management of the third stage of labour is highly effective at preventing PPH. For women delivering by C/S, Syntocinon® 5 U should be administered by slow IV injection (caution should be exercised in women with major cardiovascular disorders). Syntometrine® may be used in the absence of hypertension or cardiac disease. Misoprostol, 400 micrograms in powdered form sublingually or 600 micrograms orally (unlicensed), may be used in settings where oxytocin is not available. Women at high risk of PPH should be ideally cared for by professionals with appropriate knowledge, skills, and experience and in settings with appropriate facilities, including blood transfusion.

Clinical management

Once major PPH has been identified, management involves four components, all of which must be undertaken simultaneously:

- Communication
- Resuscitation
- Monitoring
- Investigation
- Arresting the bleeding.

Communication aims to ensure prompt and effective management of this obstetric emergency. Team approach, involving midwives, obstetricians, anaesthetists, blood transfusion personnel, theatre staff, and porters, is recommended. Resuscitation should follow a structured approach of airway, breathing, and circulation management.

Consider transferring the patient to theatre in a timely manner, as this will facilitate surgical intervention. A scribe is necessary to maintain a contemporaneous record of events. Keep the patient and partner informed. Consider transfer to ITU once the bleeding is controlled or monitoring at HDU on delivery suite, if appropriate.

Minor PPH is usually well tolerated and requires minimal intervention. Secondary PPH is due to retained placental tissue or endometritis; treatment is with antibiotics or careful evacuation of the uterus.

Common pitfalls

Blood loss is commonly underestimated, particularly when it occurs insidiously. Concealed haemorrhage, such as intraperitoneal bleeding or deep pelvic haematoma, can present a diagnostic challenge and should be considered in the differential diagnosis of post-partum collapse.

Further reading

http://www.who.int/entity/bulletin/volumes/87/3/08-052597/en/ - 52k

Prendiville WJ, Elbourne D, McDonald S (2000). Active versus expectant management in the third stage of labour. *Cochrane Database of Systematic Reviews*, **3**, CD000007.

Royal College of Obstetricians and Gynaecologists (2009). *Prevention and management of postpartum haemorrhage*. Green-top guideline No. 52. Available at: <http://www.rcog.org.uk/files/rcog-corp/GT52PostpartumHaemorrhage0411.pdf>.

Key information for post-partum haemorrhage

Major PPH
All four components must be performed simultaneously

Communication
Major PPH is an obstetric emergency

Call for help:
Midwives
Obstetricians
Anaesthetist
Porter

Inform:
Blood bank
Theatre staff
Haematologist

Regular drills and skills for all maternity staff

Resuscitation
Position patient flat
ABC approach
Anaesthetist to manage airway and guide fluid replacement
100% O_2 via face mask
10–15 L/min
14-gauge cannulae x 2
Rapid warmed infusion of fluids
Crystalloid up to 2 L
Colloid 1–2 L
Blood transfusion as soon as possible (crossmatched or uncrossmatched group-specific or 'O RhD-negative' blood)
Coagulation factor support with advice of haematologist
Keep patient warm

Monitoring and investigation
Crossmatch blood (4 U minimum)
FBC, coagulation studies, renal and liver function
Monitor temperature
Continuous pulse, BP recording, and respiratory rate (with oximeter, electrocardiogram, and automated BP recording)
Foley catheter to monitor urine output
Consider arterial line monitoring
Consider transfer to intensive therapy unit once the bleeding is controlled or at high dependency unit on delivery suite
Maintain a fluid balance chart
Documentation of interventions and their sequence
Debriefing of patient and partner

Arresting the bleeding
Massage the uterus
Bimanual uterine compression

Pharmacological options
Ergometrine 500 micrograms IM or slow IV injection (contraindicated in women with hypertension and cardiac disease)
Ergometrine 500 micrograms with oxytocin 5 U (Syntometrine®) IM injection
Misoprostol 1,000 micrograms rectally (unlicensed)
Syntocinon® 5 U slow IV injection
Syntocinon® infusion 10 IU hourly
Carboprost 250 micrograms IM every 15 min (maximum 8 doses, contraindicated in women with asthma)
Carboprost 250 micrograms may be administered by intramyometrial injection (unlicensed use)

Surgical options
Remove retained placental tissue
Repair genital tract trauma
Intrauterine balloon tamponade Haemostatic brace suturing
Bilateral ligation of uterine arteries or internal iliac arteries
Selective arterial embolization, Caesarean hysterectomy
Correct uterine inversion, if present

Post-partum psychosis

Key learning points
Three main clinical scenarios exist
Maternal mental health problems not confined to the puerperium
Need to check for pre-existing risk factors
Management in a team-based specialist setting for severe cases mandatory.

Childbirth is an event which involves physiological and psychological adaptation for the mother. Post-partum psychosis, despite the terminology, is not confined to the puerperium. It may occur antenatally and perpetuate to the puerperium.

There are three clinical syndromes:

- Maternity blues
- Post-natal depression
- Puerperal psychosis.

Maternity blues

Also known as baby blues, this affects 50–70% of women. It is a transient, self-limiting condition that most commonly starts 3–5 days after delivery and may persist for up to 2 weeks. The patient may be anxious, irritable, tearful, and down in spirits.

The pathogenesis is unknown, but the following factors may be involved:

- Declining oestrogen and progesterone levels
- An inability to cope with the sudden overwhelming change in circumstances
- Pain
- Feelings of inadequacy
- Breastfeeding
- Meeting the demands of the baby and expectations of family members.

Management centres on reassurance and social/family support. If the condition persists, the patient should be referred for psychiatric evaluation.

Post-natal depression

This can affect up to 10% of mothers. It can occur any time from conception to within 1 year of delivery. It may follow miscarriage, termination of pregnancy, live birth, or stillbirth. Symptoms include:

- Depression
- Suicidal thoughts
- Loss of appetite
- Lack of energy
- Lack of general interest
- Insomnia
- Poor concentration
- Diminished self-confidence
- Low sexual interest.

The patient may be irritable and short-tempered and harbour negative feelings about her child. Post-natal depression should be taken seriously and managed appropriately in time, not only in maternal interest, but also to avoid the infant's developmental problems. NICE (UK) recommends screening for depression in pregnant women both antenatally and at 4–6 weeks and 3–4 months post-natally. Mild to moderate depression may respond to self-help strategies and non-directive counselling. Severe depression will require antidepressants and/or psychotherapy. There is a high recurrence rate and 70% lifetime risk of depressive illness.

Puerperal psychosis

This occurs in 1–2 out of 1000 deliveries and is defined as major depression with psychotic features, for example:

- Delusions
- Hallucinations
- Gross abnormalities of speech and behaviour.

Women usually present within the first 2 weeks following the delivery. There is also the risk of suicide or infanticide in up to 5% patients. It may recur with each subsequent pregnancy. There may be a history of:

- Premorbid personality
- Psychiatric disorders
  - Schizophrenia
  - Bipolar disorders in the past or family
  - Previous episode of puerperal psychosis
- Marital problems
- Lack of family support.

High-risk patients should be referred to specialist perinatal mental health service antenatally so that an appropriate care plan can be developed and the use of prophylactic medication can be considered soon after delivery. Management includes assessing the severity of the condition, providing emotional support and counselling, and referring the patient to a psychiatrist and support groups. Ideally, the mother should be in a specialist mother-baby unit where the maternal-infant relationship can be protected. If the condition is severe, the patient will require psychotropic medications (antidepressants, antipsychotics, or mood stabilizers) for at least 6 months and, in some cases, electroconvulsive therapy (ECT). Most patients make a full recovery, but recurrence rates are high (60–80%) in the long term.

Further reading

National Institute for Health and Clinical Excellence (2007). *Antenatal and postnatal mental health: clinical management and service guidance.* NICE clinical guideline 45. Available at: <http://www.nice.org.uk/nicemedia/live/11004/30433/30433.pdf>.

Algorithm for post-partum psychosis

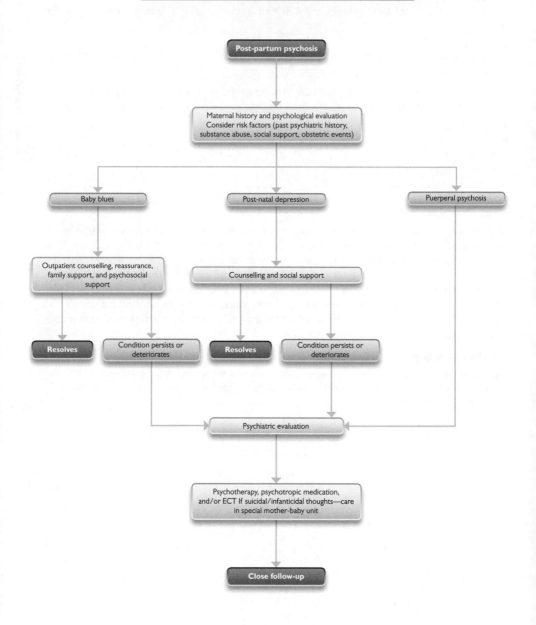

Post-partum bladder problems

Key learning points

Early identification and catheterization of women with urinary retention is vital to prevent long-term morbidity

All women should have passed urine within 6 h of delivery

Long-term catheterization or intermittent self-catheterization are helpful in the restoration of normal bladder function.

Introduction

Post-partum bladder problems include voiding dysfunction/urinary retention, UTIs, and urinary incontinence (UI).

Voiding dysfunction

Aetiology

The aetiology of post-partum voiding dysfunction and urinary retention involves physiological, neurological, and mechanical causes, including:

1. Regional anaesthesia (causing bladder overdistension injury)
2. Prolonged labour
3. Instrumental deliveries
4. Vulval trauma or vaginal haematoma, causing pain or mechanical obstruction
5. Primiparity
6. Increased birthweight.

Assessment

Symptoms and signs of voiding dysfunction range from a complete inability to void to large post-void residual volumes with no other symptoms. Clinical suspicion should be raised in patients with small voided volumes, urinary frequency, slow or intermittent stream, strain to void, incomplete bladder emptying, urgency, bladder pain or abdominal discomfort, urinary overflow incontinence, and no sensation to void.

The diagnosis of overt voiding dysfunction can be made if the patient has been unable to void within 6 h of delivery and requires catheterization to drain greater than a normal bladder capacity (400–600 mL).

The diagnosis of covert voiding dysfunction involves the inability to pass >50% of normal bladder capacity or if the post-void residual volume is >150 mL.

Management

No patient should be left for >6 h without voiding or being catheterized for residual volumes. If urine has not been passed within 6 h after birth, measures to aid voiding include:

- Effective analgesia
- Ice packs to the perineum to reduce oedema
- Mobilization of the patient to stand and walk to the toilet
- A warm bath
- Avoidance of constipation.

If urinary retention is suspected:

- The progress and management of labour should be reviewed
- Clinical examination should include abdominal palpation to check for height of bladder and vaginal inspection/examination for evidence of vulval and vaginal trauma

- If measures to encourage micturition are not successful, catheterization is indicated. Catheterization offers the most accurate post-void residual volume measurement in the post-partum period, as ultrasound measurements of residual volumes can be inaccurate because of the size of the post-partum uterus
- Fluid intake and output, as well as timing of voids and voided volumes, should be documented, using a chart
- An indwelling catheter should be used for 24 or 48 h
- Antibiotics, following a urine sample for cultures, should be considered if recatheterization is needed
- After removal of the catheter, the mother should be encouraged to pass urine every 4 h and have a strict fluid balance chart. If she is not able to pass urine in 4 h or passes <150 mL, then residual urine volumes should be checked by catheterization, and, if they are >150 mL, a catheter should be left *in situ* for 24 h, followed by further review
- Should the next trial of void be unsuccessful, an indwelling catheter should be inserted for approximately 1 week
- A repeat trial of void is undertaken a week later, and, if unsuccessful again, the patient should be instructed to perform timed voids every 3–4 h and taught intermittent self-catheterization. Monitoring of signs and symptoms of a UTI is important
- Persistent cases of voiding dysfunction should have a repeat assessment and uroflowmetry study every 2–4 weeks until complete resolution of symptoms
- Any cases that remain unresolved by 3 months require complete urodynamic investigations and management by a urogynaecologist.

Prognosis

If managed appropriately, the majority of women with voiding difficulties will have resumed normal voiding function at the time of discharge from hospital. However, failure to diagnose and manage voiding difficulties may result in chronic voiding dysfunction, requiring long-term catheterization. Residual volumes >700–750 mL at diagnosis are associated with a poorer prognosis.

Post-partum UTIs

Signs and symptoms

Symptoms of UTI in the post-partum woman are commonly dysuria, frequency of micturition, and loin/lower abdominal pain.

Treatment

If apyrexial:
    Obtain an MSU and dipstick for protein, leucocytes, blood, and nitrites
    Send urine for microscopy, culture, and sensitivity (M, C, &S) tests
    Consider antibiotics if dipstick is positive for protein, leucocytes, blood, and nitrites
If pyrexial (>38°C):
    FBC, U + Es, CRP
    IV access and obtain blood cultures
    Obtain an MSU and dipstick for protein, leucocytes, blood, and nitrites
    Send urine for M, C, & S
    Analgesia and broad-spectrum antibiotics should be commenced.

Post-partum urinary incontinence

The reported prevalence of UI in the post-partum period is approximately 30% in the first 3 months. Stress incontinence is more common than urgency incontinence among post-partum women, especially in primiparas ones. Women with post-partum incontinence generally have low frequency of symptoms.

Management

- MSU analysis to exclude infection
- For severe symptoms—exclude the possibility of an early vesico-vaginal or ureteric-vaginal (post-C/S) fistula (rare)

- Pelvic floor exercises are recommended, as they are known to reduce the risk of long-term incontinence problems
- Women with involuntary leakage of urine, which does not resolve or becomes worse, should be evaluated.

Further reading

Lim JL (2010). Post-partum voiding dysfunction and urinary retention. *Australian and New Zealand Journal of Obstetrics and Gynaecology*, **50**, 502–5.

National Institute for Health and Clinical Excellence (2006). *Routine postnatal care of women and their babies.* NICE clinical guideline 37. Available at: <http://www.nice.org.uk/nicemedia/pdf/CG37NICEguideline.pdf>.

Care pathways for post-partum bladder problems

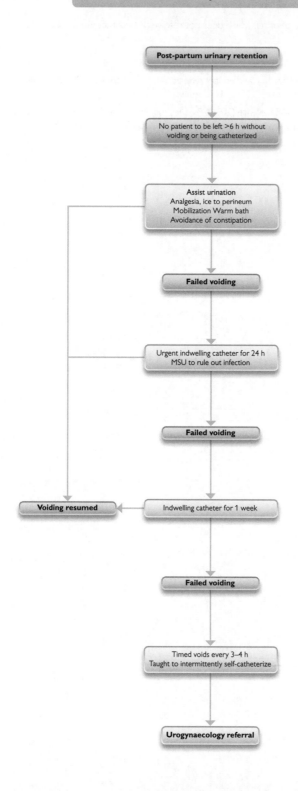

Care pathways for post-partum bladder problems

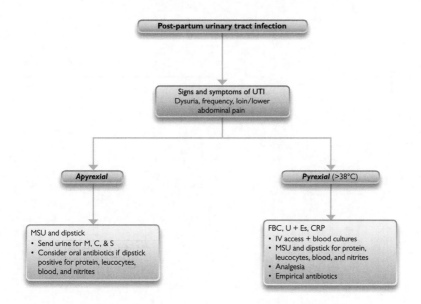

Post-partum urinary tract infection

Signs and symptoms of UTI
Dysuria, frequency, loin/lower abdominal pain

Apyrexial

Pyrexial (>38°C)

MSU and dipstick
- Send urine for M, C, & S
- Consider oral antibiotics if dipstick positive for protein, leucocytes, blood, and nitrites

FBC, U + Es, CRP
- IV access + blood cultures
- MSU and dipstick for protein, leucocytes, blood, and nitrites
- Analgesia
- Empirical antibiotics

Care pathways for post-partum bladder problems

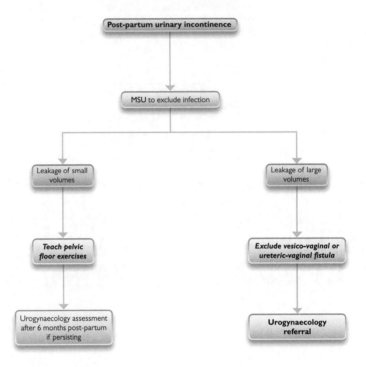

Post-partum urinary incontinence

↓

MSU to exclude infection

Leakage of small volumes	Leakage of large volumes
↓	↓
Teach pelvic floor exercises	*Exclude vesico-vaginal or ureteric-vaginal fistula*
↓	↓
Urogynaecology assessment after 6 months post-partum if persisting	**Urogynaecology referral**

Management of perineal tears

Key learning points

Classification of tears from first degree to fourth degree
Type of surgical technique for repair of tears standardized
Follow-up vital to reduce morbidity.

Introduction

In the UK, 38% of women sustain some form of perineal tear after vaginal delivery.

The following classification has been adopted by the International Consultation on Incontinence and the RCOG.

First degree:
 Injury to perineal skin only
Second degree:
 Injury to perineum, involving perineal muscles but not involving the anal sphincter
Third degree:
 Injury to perineum, involving the anal sphincter complex:
  3a: < 50% of external anal sphincter (EAS) thickness torn
  3b: >50% of EAS thickness torn
  3c: both EAS and internal anal sphincter (IAS) torn
Fourth degree:
 Injury to perineum, involving the anal sphincter complex (EAS and IAS) and anal epithelium.

Management

All women having a vaginal delivery who have sustained a perineal tear should be examined to assess the severity of damage.

Following first or second degree perineal tears, the skin may be left unsutured to reduce pain and dyspareunia. Most second-degree tears require suturing to achieve normalization of the perineal anatomy.

Following third or fourth degree perineal tears, the EAS should be repaired, either with an overlapping or end-to-end method. If the IAS is torn, this should be repaired separately with interrupted sutures. Repair should be performed in an operating theatre, under regional or general anaesthesia.

Repair of the EAS muscle should be performed, with either monofilament sutures, such as 3-0 polydioxanone (PDS), or polyglactin (Vicryl®). For repair of the IAS muscle, a fine-suture gauge, such as 3-0 PDS and 2-0 Vicryl®, should be used.

Post-operatively, broad-spectrum antibiotics and laxatives should be used to reduce the incidence of post-operative infections and wound dehiscence. Physiotherapy and follow-up are recommended.

Women who have had obstetric anal sphincter repair should be reviewed 6–12 weeks post-partum by a multidisciplinary team who have special interest clinics for post-natal pelvic floor problems. Endoanal ultrasonography and anorectal manometry should be offered to evaluate sphincter anatomy and function.

Symptomatic women or women with abnormal anorectal manometric or endoanal ultrasonographic features should be offered an elective C/S for their future delivery. Prognosis following EAS repair is very good, and 60–80% women are asymptomatic at 12 months.

Further reading

Department of Health (2005). Government Statistical Service. *NHS Maternity Statistics*.

Gordon B, Mackrodt C, Fern E, Truesdale A, Ayers S, Grant A (1998). The Ipswich Childbirth Study: 1. A randomised evaluation of two stage postpartum perineal repair leaving the skin unsutured. *British Journal of Obstetrics and Gynaecology*, **105**, 435–40.

Revicky V, Nirmal D, Mukhopadhyay S, Morris EP, Nieto JJ (2010). Could a mediolateral episiotomy prevent obstetric anal sphincter injury? *European Journal of Obstetrics & Gynecology and Reproductive Biology*, **150**, 142–6.

Royal College of Obstetricians and Gynaecologists (2007). *The management of third- and fourth-degree perineal tears*. Green-top guideline No. 29. Available at: <http://www.rcog.org.uk/files/rcog-corp/GTG2911022011.pdf>.

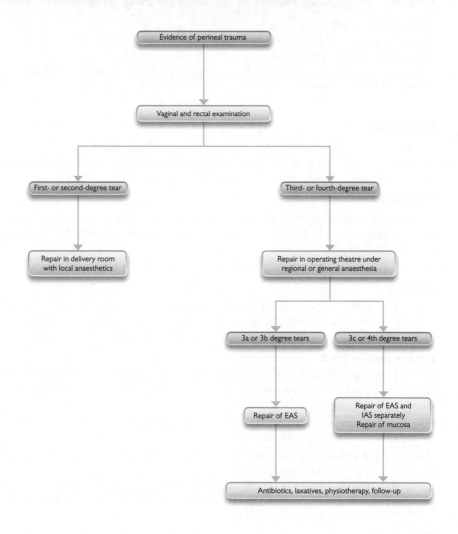

Care pathway for the management of perineal tears

Evidence of perineal trauma

Vaginal and rectal examination

First- or second-degree tear

Repair in delivery room with local anaesthetics

Third- or fourth-degree tear

Repair in operating theatre under regional or general anaesthesia

3a or 3b degree tears

3c or 4th degree tears

Repair of EAS

Repair of EAS and IAS separately
Repair of mucosa

Antibiotics, laxatives, physiotherapy, follow-up

Puerperal abdominal distension

Key learning points
Causes of abdominal distension very heterogeneous

Need to identify severe illness early

Management depends on underlying cause, but, if sepsis suspected, instigate rapid treatment with a sepsis bundle.

Introduction
Puerperal abdominal distension can have a very heterogeneous pathophysiology.

Causes of abdominal swelling may be simple, as a constipation and diastasis of abdominal muscles, or more serious as puerperal sepsis, ileus, bowel obstruction, Ogilvie syndrome, or severe haemorrhage.

Management
Management of puerperal abdominal distension largely depends on the underlying cause. Post-partum constipation can be overcome by increased fluid intake and laxatives. Diastasis of abdominal muscles may improve after physiotherapy.

More serious causes of puerperal abdominal distension require timely diagnosis and treatment.

Infection
Puerperal sepsis is a life-threatening condition and, therefore, requires a multidisciplinary approach, with immediate administration of antibiotics, using a 'sepsis bundle' approach, before further exploration of diagnostic possibilities. Early involvement of an anaesthetist and admission to HDU may be necessary.

Gastrointestinal tract
Paralytic ileus is a rare complication of a normal vaginal birth; however, it can occur following C/S. Main symptoms are absent bowel sounds and abdominal distension. Gastric decompression, IV fluid, and exclusion of oral intake may be required.

Bowel obstruction can occur mainly following C/S. Main symptoms are abdominal distension, nausea, vomiting, and abdominal pain. Early surgical involvement and laparotomy may be necessary.

Ogilvie syndrome is the acute pseudo-obstruction and dilatation of the colon in the absence of any mechanical obstruction and can occur following normal or Caesarean birth. Colonic pseudo-obstruction is characterized by massive dilatation of the caecum and right colon. It usually resolves with conservative therapy, after stopping oral ingestions and an NGT, but may require colonoscopic decompression. It is a serious medical disorder, and the mortality rate can be as high as 30%.

Blood loss
Acute haemorrhage may develop rapidly, following Caesarean birth, due to a complication of haemostasis. In this case, abdominal distension has a rapid onset and is accompanied by deteriorating vital signs, mainly tachycardia, tachypnoea, and hypotension. Rapid recognition, senior involvement, and timely relaparotomy may be crucial.

Further reading
Dua A and Onyeka BA (2006). Ogilvie syndrome complicated by caecal perforation in a post-Caesarean section patient: a case report. *The Internet Journal of Gynecology and Obstetrics*, **5**, No. 2.

Irwin RS and Rippe JM (2003). *Intensive care medicine*. Lippincott Williams & Wilkins, Philadelphia and London (ISBN 0-7817-3548-3).

Laskin MD, Tessler K, Kives S (2009). Cecal perforation due to paralytic ileus following primary caesarean section. *Journal of Obstetrics and Gynaecology Canada*, **31**, 167–71.

Leg pain and swelling in pregnancy and puerperium

Key learning points

Thromboembolic disease remains a significant cause of morbidity and mortality in pregnant women

Health care systems must have guidance and policies in place to detect thrombosis early and treat appropriately

All pregnant women should be risk-assessed and thromboprophylaxis considered

Other causes for leg swelling should be excluded.

Introduction

Common causes of leg pain and swelling in pregnancy and puerperium include:

- DVT
- Superficial thrombophlebitis
- Cellulitis.

Venous thromboembolism (VTE) is the leading cause of maternal morbidity and mortality in the developed world. VTE includes DVT of the leg, calf, or pelvis and PE. The incidence of VTE in pregnancy is 1–2 in 1000 pregnancies. There is a significant risk of VTE in both antenatal and post-natal periods; however, the risk of PE is much greater in the puerperium. DVT must be ruled out in all cases of unilateral leg pain and swelling. During pregnancy, the left leg is more commonly affected than the right. The vast majority of thromboses involve the iliofemoral veins in pregnancy, and these have a higher risk of embolism to the lungs than calf vein thrombi. If the woman has had a previous VTE, there is a 5–10% risk of recurrence in subsequent pregnancies. About 10% of patients also develop a post-phlebitic leg syndrome, with persistent symptoms of swelling and pain in the affected leg.

Risks

Pregnancy itself serves as a major risk factor for the development of thrombosis. This is due to venous stasis in the lower limbs, pelvic trauma around birth, the procoagulant state of pregnancy, and suppressed fibrinolysis. Other common risk factors for the development of VTE include:

1. Previous personal or family history of VTE
2. Obesity
3. C/S or other surgery unrelated to pregnancy
4. Immobility, including prolonged hospitalization
5. Smoking
6. Presence of lupus anticoagulant
7. Severe pre-eclampsia
8. Higher maternal age
9. Air travel
10. Assisted conception
11. Thrombophilias, e.g. antithrombin III deficiency or protein C/protein S deficiency (women with previous VTE should be screened for thrombophilia before pregnancy).

Clinical diagnosis

DVT

Calf pain

Swelling of leg (usually unilateral)

Increased leg girth on measurement

Elevated skin temperature

Change of colour, i.e. increased redness of the limb

Tenderness

Pyrexia

Homan's sign positive (pain in the calf on dorsiflexion of the foot).

Lower abdominal pain is a feature of high DVT. Clinical diagnosis may be correct in only 50% of the time. Hence, an objective diagnostic test is required.

PE

Sudden-onset dyspnoea

Collapse

Chest pain

Haemoptysis

Faintness

Raised jugular venous pressure (JVP)

Focal signs in chest

Tachycardia

Tachypnoea

Evidence of DVT in the leg.

Investigations

- FBC (leucocytosis), thrombophilia screen, U + Es, LFTs, and coagulation screen
- Diagnostic imaging—ultrasound (compression or duplex), contrast venography, with shielding of the uterus, or MRI
- D-dimer levels may be elevated in normal pregnancy, so a positive test is not consistent with a diagnosis of VTE. However, if the levels of D-dimer are low, VTE is unlikely
- If PE suspected—electrocardiogram (ECG), arterial blood gases (ABGs), CXR, ventilation/perfusion (V/Q) scan or spiral CT/MRI, and bilateral duplex leg ultrasound will be needed.

Treatment

- Superficial thrombophlebitis is caused by venous stasis and should be managed with elastic supports, limb elevation, and topical analgesics
- Once VTE is suspected, treatment should be commenced while diagnostic tests are awaited
- In cases with DVT, the affected leg should be elevated and graduated elastic compression stockings applied to promote good flow via deep veins and to reduce oedema. Mobilization is recommended. If diagnostic imaging reports a low risk of VTE, yet there is high clinical suspicion, anticoagulant treatment should be continued, with repeat testing in 1 week. If repeat test gives a negative result, treatment can be discontinued
- LMWHs are the drugs of choice for the treatment of VTE. They are as effective as unfractionated heparin in pregnancy, yet safer. A twice-daily dosage regimen of LMWHs is recommended in treating VTE in pregnancy (enoxaparin 1 mg/kg bd; dalteparin 100 U/kg). Long-term users of LMWHs have a lower risk of osteoporosis and bone fractures than unfractionated heparin. The peak anti-Xa activity should be measured 3 h post-injection to ensure correct dosage (target range—0.5–1.2 IU/mL)
- Unfractionated heparin has been the traditional treatment in the initial management of VTE, including massive PE. The regimen is a loading dose of 5000 IU, followed by continuous IV infusion of 1000–2000 IU/h with an initial concentration of 1000 IU/mL. Activated partial thromboplastin time (APTT) levels should be measured 6 h after the loading dose and then on a daily basis (therapeutic target APTT ratio—1.5–2.5 times the control). Therapeutic dose anticoagulation should be continued for at least 6 months, following the VTE event. After delivery, treatment should continue for at least 6 weeks. Breastfeeding is not contraindicated in patients taking warfarin or heparin. Where DVT threatens leg viability, surgical embolectomy or thrombolytic therapy may be considered

- In cases with PE, high-flow oxygen and aggressive fluid resuscitation, along with therapeutic-dose anticoagulation, must be commenced until investigations to exclude the diagnosis have taken place. Treatment should be continued, even when ultrasound venogram and CT scan are negative or V/Q scan indicates a low probability of PE, but there is a high clinical suspicion of PE. In such cases, alternative tests (spiral CTPA/MRI/V/Q scan) or repeat testing in 1 week should be undertaken. Except in rare cases, bleeding in a post-operative woman can be managed, and thus the risk related to VTE significantly outweighs the risk of bleeding. IVC filter may be considered for recurrent PE, despite adequate anticoagulation, or if anticoagulation is contraindicated. In life-threatening massive PE, thrombolytic therapy, percutaneous catheter thrombus fragmentation, or surgical embolectomy may be required
- To avoid the risk of developing an epidural haematoma with regional anaesthesia, women receiving anticoagulation should be advised not to inject any further heparin if they think labour has started. Regional anaesthesia should be avoided until at least 12 h after the last dose of LMWH (24 h if therapeutic dose). Similarly, LMWH should not be administered for 4 h after the removal of the epidural catheter, and the catheter should not be removed within 12 h of LMWH injection.

Further reading

National Institute for Health and Clinical Excellence (2010). Venous thromboembolism: reducing the risk. Reducing the risk of venous thromboembolism (deep vein thrombosis and pulmonary embolism) in patients admitted to hospital. NICE clinical guideline 92. Available at: <http://www.nice.org.uk/nicemedia/live/12695/47195/47195.pdf>.

Royal College of Obstetricians and Gynaecologists (2007). *The acute management of thrombosis and embolism during pregnancy and the puerperium.* Green-top guideline No. 37b (reviewed 2010). Available at: <http://www.rcog.org.uk/files/rcog-corp/GTG37b_230611.pdf>.

Royal College of Obstetricians and Gynaecologists (2009). *Reducing the risk of thrombosis and embolism during pregnancy and the puerperium.* Green-top guideline No. 37a. Available at: <http://www.rcog.org.uk/files/rcog-corp/GTG37aReducingRiskThrombosis.pdf>.

Algorithm for the management of leg pain and swelling in pregnancy/puerperium

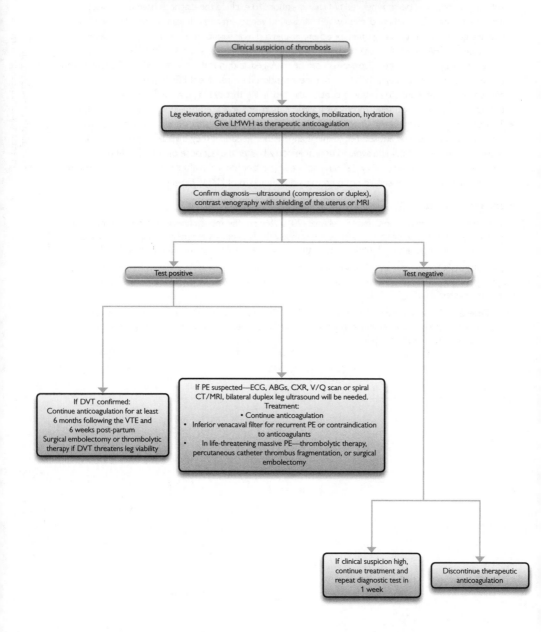

Clinical suspicion of thrombosis

Leg elevation, graduated compression stockings, mobilization, hydration
Give LMWH as therapeutic anticoagulation

Confirm diagnosis—ultrasound (compression or duplex), contrast venography with shielding of the uterus or MRI

Test positive

Test negative

If DVT confirmed:
Continue anticoagulation for at least 6 months following the VTE and 6 weeks post-partum
Surgical embolectomy or thrombolytic therapy if DVT threatens leg viability

If PE suspected—ECG, ABGs, CXR, V/Q scan or spiral CT/MRI, bilateral duplex leg ultrasound will be needed.
Treatment:
• Continue anticoagulation
• Inferior venacaval filter for recurrent PE or contraindication to anticoagulants
• In life-threatening massive PE—thrombolytic therapy, percutaneous catheter thrombus fragmentation, or surgical embolectomy

If clinical suspicion high, continue treatment and repeat diagnostic test in 1 week

Discontinue therapeutic anticoagulation

Maternal collapse

Key learning points

Summon help immediately upon encountering a maternal collapse

Local education strategy should include multidisciplinary drills and skills sessions

Following a collapse, instigate immediate supportive strategies, followed by diagnostic strategies to establish a cause.

Introduction

Collapse is a non-specific term, implying a complete or partial loss of consciousness, either as a primary cerebral event or secondary to cardiovascular problem, leading to cerebral hypoperfusion. It can range from a simple faint to a catastrophic life-threatening event.

Causes

Collapse in a pregnant woman during, or immediately after, labour is rare. The most important causes of acute collapse in pregnancy are:

- PE
- Amniotic fluid embolism
- Acute aortic dissection
- Severe pre-eclampsia
- Eclampsia
- Cerebrovascular accidents
- Sepsis
- Massive obstetric haemorrhage
- Acute coronary syndrome
- Thrombosed mechanical prosthetic heart valves
- Cardiac failure due to cardiomyopathy
- Anaesthetic complications
  - Failed intubation
  - Anaphylaxis
  - Complications of regional or local anaesthetic agents.

It is imperative that all health care professionals dealing with pregnant women are prepared for, and trained in, managing such an emergency. Obstetricians and midwives should attend local skills and drills sessions and at least basic life support training once a year.

Pregnant women develop hypoxia faster than non-pregnant women and can suffer irreversible brain damage within 4–6 min after cardiac arrest. Many physiological factors in pregnancy may impede expected response to CPR and thus need to be considered in advance. The clinical outcome of a collapse will often depend on the successful management of the first few minutes. The management is based on supporting the different organ systems that are affected.

In women who are high-risk, pre-pregnancy counselling should be offered, and, during pregnancy, a plan of antenatal care and peripartum management should be made by the appropriate multidisciplinary team.

Management

- If internal haemorrhage is suspected, the woman may need immediate laparotomy and anaesthetic/ITU involvement
- Sepsis should be aggressively managed, with appropriate fluid management, antimicrobials, and rapid identification and elimination of the possible source
- The diagnosis of PE is based on a clinical suspicion, supported by diagnostic test. LMWH is the treatment option of choice

- The management of acute coronary syndrome is based on immediate angiography and percutaneous coronary intervention. ECG, CXR, and ABGs should be performed if cardiovascular cause is suspected. There is no clinical evidence for fibrinolytic therapy as a reperfusion strategy in pregnancy, and it is best avoided, as the risk of haemorrhage outweighs the possible benefit of treatment
- Patients with a prosthetic heart valve who present with the disappearance of prosthetic heart sounds or a new murmur should receive an urgent cardiac ultrasound to rule out a thrombosed prosthetic valve. Therapeutic anticoagulation levels must be maintained in patients with mechanical prosthetic heart valves
- If intracranial pathology is suspected, cerebral imaging (CT/MRI) is needed, and neurosurgical/neurological opinion should be sought at the earliest
- A high index of suspicion is important for the diagnosis of amniotic fluid embolism in women with acute collapse. Supportive management of the different affected systems is the mainstay of management. Ventilation, inotropic support, and administration of fresh frozen plasma, cryoprecipitate, and platelets will be required. Hysterectomy may be required to control PPH. If the woman has not delivered, perimortem C/S should be performed within 5 min to aid maternal resuscitation in the face of cardiac arrest.

Steps of maternal resuscitation

A structured approach can be lifesaving (ABCDEF).

1. Primary survey
   1. Lateral tilt to relieve aortocaval compression
   2. Airway—open airway with head tilt and chin lift; a jaw thrust may be needed (to support the cervical spine)
   3. Breathing and ventilation—assess for chest movement and breath sounds, and feel for breathing. If not breathing, put out a cardiac arrest call and begin CPR
   4. Circulation—carotid pulse should be checked and circulation optimized by aggressive IV fluids and blood transfusion, if indicated; haemorrhage should be arrested
   5. Disability or neurological status assessment
   6. Environmental control—to avoid injury and hypothermia, and ensure safety of woman and staff
   7. Fetus—once maternal condition is stable, assess fetal well-being and plan delivery as appropriate.
   8. Reversible causes of collapse, such as hypoxia, hypovolaemia, hypo- and hyperkalaemia/metabolic, hyperthermia, tension pneumothorax, tamponade (cardiac), toxins, thrombosis (coronary or pulmonary), should be considered and treated as necessary
2. Secondary survey
   1. Once the life-threatening conditions have been found and dealt with in the primary survey, a systematic assessment of other organ systems from head to toe (head, neck, chest, abdomen, pelvis, limbs, internal examinations) should follow. A good-quality history should be obtained from the patient or any witnesses.
   2. Ongoing monitoring should include: heart rate/ECG, BP, pulse oximetry, respiration, temperature, urine output, and fetal heart monitoring where appropriate. Bloods should be sent for: FBC, coagulation profile, U + Es, LFTs, G & S or crossmatch, and blood glucose
3. Definitive care should follow, involving a multidisciplinary team of relevant specialists.

Further reading

Royal College of Obstetricians and Gynaecologists (2011). *Maternal collapse in pregnancy and the puerperium.* Green-top guideline No. 56. Available at: <http://www.rcog.org.uk/files/rcog-corp/GTG56.pdf>.

Algorithms for maternal collapse

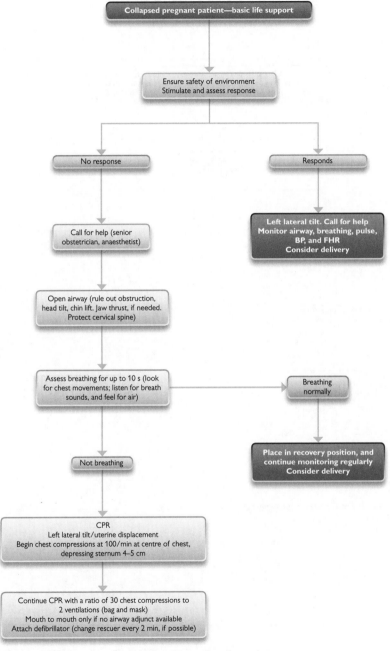

Collapsed pregnant patient—basic life support

Ensure safety of environment
Stimulate and assess response

No response

Responds

Left lateral tilt. Call for help
Monitor airway, breathing, pulse,
BP, and FHR
Consider delivery

Call for help (senior
obstetrician, anaesthetist)

Open airway (rule out obstruction,
head tilt, chin lift. Jaw thrust, if needed.
Protect cervical spine)

Assess breathing for up to 10 s (look
for chest movements; listen for breath
sounds, and feel for air)

Breathing
normally

Place in recovery position, and
continue monitoring regularly
Consider delivery

Not breathing

CPR
Left lateral tilt/uterine displacement
Begin chest compressions at 100/min at centre of chest,
depressing sternum 4–5 cm

Continue CPR with a ratio of 30 chest compressions to
2 ventilations (bag and mask)
Mouth to mouth only if no airway adjunct available
Attach defibrillator (change rescuer every 2 min, if possible)

Adapted with kind permission from the Resuscitation Council.

Algorithms for maternal collapse

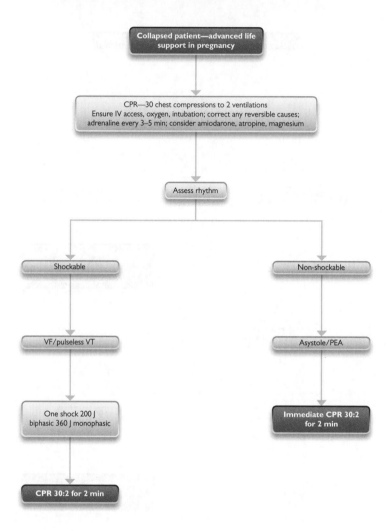

Adapted with kind permission from the Resuscitation Council.

Instrumental delivery

Key learning points

Instrumental delivery useful to expedite delivery or to aid the exhausted mother

Consider indications and contraindications carefully

Obtain verbal or written consent for delivery and episiotomy

Perform under appropriate analgesia/anaesthesia.

Introduction

Instrumental delivery is often an alternative to emergency C/S. The aim is to achieve vaginal delivery, with minimal maternal and neonatal morbidity. Knowledge of pelvic anatomy and competency in the assessment of the baby are important prerequisites. The operator must be competent in the use of the chosen instrument. The forceps and vacuum extractor (ventouse) are the only two available options. A posterior cup where the suction tubing does not interfere with the placement of the cup on the fetal flexion point (metal or rigid plastic) or Kielland's forceps are preferred for rotational deliveries. Any suitable forceps or vacuum device can be used for traction, only when the head is in occipitoanterior position and at station + 1 or below.

Forceps

- Made of metal and consist of four major components:
  - Handle
  - Lock
  - Shank
  - Blades.

Vacuum extractors

- Made of metal or plastic (flexible or rigid)—a metal posterior and rigid plastic anterior cup are shown.
- Five or 6 cm in diameter.

Indications

- Presumed fetal compromise
- Failure to progress in the second stage
- Maternal exhaustion
- Hypertensive crisis
- Cardiac disease class III or IV (New York Heart Association classification)
- Myasthenia gravis
- Spinal cord injury
- Forceps may be used for aftercoming head in breech presentation.

Contraindications

- Mother declines consent
- Head 2/5 or more palpable
- Leading bony edge of the skull above the ishial spines
- Excessive moulding
- Malpresentation
- Vacuum extraction contraindicated below 34 weeks' gestation. Cautious use between 34 and 36 weeks.

The relative merits of vacuum extraction and forceps

Vacuum extraction, compared with forceps, is:

More likely to fail at achieving a vaginal delivery

More likely to be associated with a cephalhaematoma

More likely to be associated with a retinal haemorrhage

More likely to be associated with maternal worries about baby

Less likely to be associated with significant maternal vaginal or perineal trauma

No more likely to be associated with delivery by C/S

No more likely to be associated with low 5-min Apgar scores

No more likely to be associated with the need for phototherapy.

Further reading

Johanson RB and Menon V (1999). Vacuum extraction versus forceps for assisted vaginal delivery. *Cochrane Database of Systematic Reviews*, **2**, CD000224.

Care pathway for instrumental deliveries

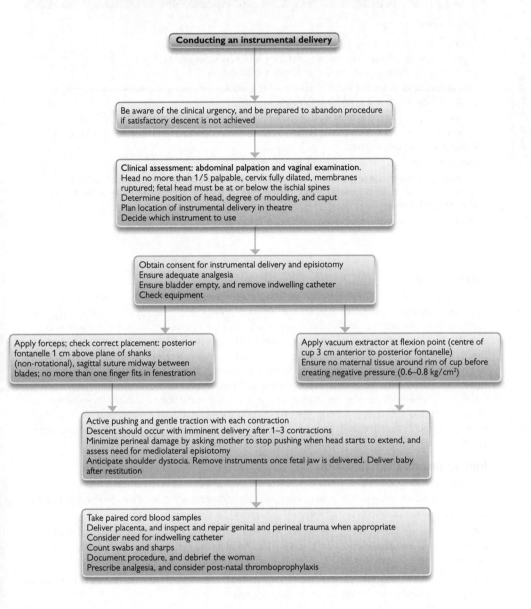

Conducting an instrumental delivery

Be aware of the clinical urgency, and be prepared to abandon procedure if satisfactory descent is not achieved

Clinical assessment: abdominal palpation and vaginal examination.
Head no more than 1/5 palpable, cervix fully dilated, membranes ruptured; fetal head must be at or below the ischial spines
Determine position of head, degree of moulding, and caput
Plan location of instrumental delivery in theatre
Decide which instrument to use

Obtain consent for instrumental delivery and episiotomy
Ensure adequate analgesia
Ensure bladder empty, and remove indwelling catheter
Check equipment

Apply forceps; check correct placement: posterior fontanelle 1 cm above plane of shanks (non-rotational), sagittal suture midway between blades; no more than one finger fits in fenestration

Apply vacuum extractor at flexion point (centre of cup 3 cm anterior to posterior fontanelle)
Ensure no maternal tissue around rim of cup before creating negative pressure (0.6–0.8 kg/cm²)

Active pushing and gentle traction with each contraction
Descent should occur with imminent delivery after 1–3 contractions
Minimize perineal damage by asking mother to stop pushing when head starts to extend, and assess need for mediolateral episiotomy
Anticipate shoulder dystocia. Remove instruments once fetal jaw is delivered. Deliver baby after restitution

Take paired cord blood samples
Deliver placenta, and inspect and repair genital and perineal trauma when appropriate
Consider need for indwelling catheter
Count swabs and sharps
Document procedure, and debrief the woman
Prescribe analgesia, and consider post-natal thromboprophylaxis

Emergency Caesarean section

Key learning points

C/S rates are increasing

Improvements in anaesthesia, blood transfusion, antibiotics, surgical techniques, and thromboprophylaxis have combined to increase the safety of C/S

Prophylactic antibiotics and perioperative thromboprophylaxis (hydration, early mobilization, graduated stockings, and LMWH) are recommended

Regional anaesthesia is the technique of choice

Informed consent, G & S for blood, bladder catheterization, antacids, H2 receptor blockers are important preoperative steps

Location of placenta should be identified prior to any C/S

Good surgical technique and adherence to guidelines/standard of care are essential during the surgery to prevent complications. Senior help should be sought, without any delay or hesitation, in case difficulties arise

Women should have the opportunity to discuss future pregnancies after C/S.

Introduction

Almost a quarter of all deliveries in the UK are currently performed by C/S, but the rates of this procedure vary widely throughout the world, depending on patient population, local resources, and labour ward protocols. Concerns have been raised over the surgical and future reproductive implications of rising rates of C/S. Sequelae of vaginal birth, such as pelvic floor damage, maternal choice, complex and older obstetric patients, litigious environment, and avoidance of potentially difficult instrumental deliveries, are some of the factors contributing to these trends. The number of difficult Caesareans is also increasing due to a rise in the rate of repeat C/S and the presence of associated medical conditions such as obesity.

C/S may be performed as an elective or emergency procedure, but the latter is associated with higher rates of complications and morbidity. Although the majority of C/S are performed for maternal or fetal indications; some may be performed at maternal request without medical reason—this area of practice remains controversial, with differences of opinion amongst individual obstetricians.

Indications and classification

The indications for over 70% of procedures are failure to progress in labour, suspected fetal compromise, breech presentation, and repeat C/S. To ensure standardized data reporting and clear communication within teams, C/S are now classified into four categories, depending on the urgency of situation.

Category 1—immediate threat to the life of the woman or fetus, e.g. placental abruption, cord prolapse, uterine rupture, fetal bradycardia, or FBS pH <7.20. The aim is to deliver the baby as rapidly as possible (decision-to-delivery interval of 30 min or less) but without endangering the mother.

Category 2—maternal or fetal compromise which is not immediately life-threatening, e.g. APH or failure to progress in labour with some maternal or fetal compromise.

Category 3—no maternal or fetal compromise but needs early delivery.

Category 4—at a time to suit the woman and maternity services (elective).

A full informed written consent must be gained from the mother prior to any C/S; however, this may not be practical in some category 1 emergency C/S. In such circumstances, verbal consent should be obtained and clearly documented in the notes.

Classification reproduced from Lucas DN, Yentis SM, Kinsella SM et al., 'Urgency of caesarean section: a new classification', *Journal of the Royal Society of Medicine*, **93**, pp. 346–350, copyright 2000, with permission from SAGE Publications.

Preoperative preparation

The operating surgeon should have full knowledge of the patient's obstetric and medical history as well as the indication for the procedure. It is essential to identify the location of the placenta prior to the C/S. If it is known to be low-lying, then a senior obstetrician and senior anaesthetist should be present in theatre. Blood should be crossmatched and available, and the patient should have been informed about the risk of bleeding and the need for surgical procedures, including hysterectomy, if needed.

It is good practice to check the FBC to rule out anaemia and G & S in case blood is required during or after the surgery in all cases. H2 receptor antagonists or a proton pump inhibitor should be administered preoperatively to reduce the gastric acid content in case of need for general anaesthesia. This, along with the use of a cuffed endotracheal tube, decreases the risk of aspiration of gastric contents in the mother (Mendelson's syndrome). A urethral catheter should be inserted to ensure the bladder is empty. Regional anaesthesia (spinal or epidural) is the technique of choice. Neonatologist should be present in the theatre.

Intraoperative technique

The mother should be positioned supine, with a 15° lateral tilt, to avoid venacaval compression. Shaving should be avoided or, if required, should be done immediately prior to the surgery. Prophylactic antibiotics just before skin incision have been shown to substantially reduce infectious morbidity, and either ampicillin or cephalosporin may be used.

Transverse suprapubic (Pfannenstiel or Joel Cohen) skin incisions are widely used, and the lower segment uterine incision is the standard approach. Before an incision is made, the rotation of the uterus should be noted and corrected, if possible. In cases of obstructed labour, the uterovesical fold of the peritoneum may be located higher and the peritoneum should be opened higher up to avoid bladder injury. When difficulties in delivering the presenting part arise, an extension of the transverse uterine incision in the shape of a 'J' or an inverted 'T' may be required. There are few indications for a classical C/S such as preterm delivery with poorly formed lower segment, poor lower segment with transverse lie, transverse lie with fetal back presenting, previous classical section, cervical fibroid, or carcinoma of the cervix.

Occasionally, if the fetal head is high, making delivery difficult, Wrigley's forceps can be applied to accomplish the delivery. Similarly, in the second stage, the fetal head may be impacted deep into the pelvis. Delivery may be accomplished by asking an assistant to push the head up from below, or the use of a tocolytic (e.g. terbutaline) may help to relax the uterus, particularly when the membranes have ruptured. Rarely, the fetus may need to be delivered by the breech first to enable disimpaction of the head.

Administration of oxytocin and application of controlled cord traction should be used for delivering the placenta. Routine manual removal of the placenta is not recommended, as it often leads to increased blood loss and risk of infection. The uterine cavity should be inspected to ensure complete removal of placenta and membranes. The uterus may be repaired *in situ* or following exteriorization which is helpful in case of extension of the incision. The angles of the uterine wound are identified, and the lower segment should be sutured in two layers, using a continuous absorbable suture. Non-closure of the peritoneum saves operating time and is associated with less post-operative morbidity and requirement of analgesia. The rectus sheath should be closed with continuous absorbable suture (1 cm from the edge and 1 cm apart). Although not routinely necessary, a fat stitch may be used if the fat layer is >2 cm thick. Closure of skin is often performed, based on the surgeon's choice of suture material/staples.

It is a good practice to set up or continue oxytocin infusion for 4–6 h, following the delivery, to facilitate uterine contraction, especially in women who have had overdistended uteri (big baby, twins) or a long labour with inadequate uterine activity. Following the procedure, clear documentation of the operative steps and debriefing to the patient are essential, clearly identifying any difficulties encountered or complications with the surgery. A plan for management of subsequent deliveries should be included.

Further reading

Baskett TF, Calder AA, Arulkumaran S (2007). Caesarean section. In *Munro Kerr's operative obstetrics*, 11th edn, pp. 155–66. Elsevier Saunders, London.

Bonney EA and Myers JE (2011). Caesarean section: techniques and complications. *Obstetrics, Gynaecology & Reproductive Medicine*, **21**, 97–102.

National Institute for Health and Clinical Excellence (2011). *Caesarean section*. NICE clinical guideline 132. Available at: <http://www.nice.org.uk/nicemedia/live/13620/57163/57163.pdf>.

Care pathway for emergency Caesarean section

- Confirm the indication
- Classify category (1 to 4), and plan timing of delivery accordingly
- A full informed written consent (verbal consent in category 1)
- Identify the location of the placenta (involve senior team and crossmatch blood in case of low-lying)
- Perform surgical checklist

- Check FBC and G & S
- H2 receptor antagonists or a proton pump inhibitor and antacid
- Urethral catheter
- Appropriate anaesthesia
- Neonatologist present in the theatre

Indications for a classical Caesarean section:
- Preterm delivery with poorly formed lower segment
- Poor lower segment with transverse lie
- Transverse lie with fetal back presenting
- Previous classical section
- Cervical fibroid or cervical carcinoma

- Mother positioned supine with a 15 degree lateral tilt
- Prophylactic antibiotics
- Transverse suprapubic skin incision and lower segment uterine incision
- If difficulties with delivery—extension of uterine incision in the shape of a 'J' or an inverted 'T'
- Deliver placenta by controlled cord traction
- Check cavity is empty
- Lower segment should be sutured in two layers, using a continuous absorbable suture

- Consider prophylactic oxytocin infusion for 4–6 h
- Clear documentation of the operative steps
- Debrief the patient

Key learning points

Regular observation of vital signs, including vaginal blood loss, is essential in the immediate post-operative period at the recovery area

Early warning charts should be used for early detection and timely management of complications

Consider thromboprophylaxis measures

Breastfeeding should be encouraged as early as possible

Patients with suspected infection will require aggressive antibiotic therapy.

Introduction

When compared to vaginal delivery, Caesarean delivery is associated with increased risk of VTE, abdominal pain, injury to bowel/bladder, need for hysterectomy, and maternal death. The major threats to the young, otherwise healthy, women undergoing C/S arise from haemorrhage, anaesthetic problems, sepsis, urinary tract injuries, and thromboembolism.

Post-operative management

For immediate post-operative management, please follow the Algorithm. Some important issues are highlighted below.

1. **Blood loss**—besides vital parameters, attention should be paid to vaginal blood loss, level of uterine fundus, temperature, and urinary output

2. **Diet and fluid intake**—women who are recovering well from the operation and do not have complications can eat and drink when they feel hungry or thirsty. In women requiring longer periods of IV fluid therapy, e.g. those with renal disease, medical problems, or bowel complications, adjustments may be made in the fluid regime to maintain adequate fluid balance. In such situations, serum electrolytes should be checked and any imbalances corrected appropriately

3. **Urine output**—at least 30 mL/h of urinary output must be maintained. If less, the patient may be hypotensive, dehydrated, or the ureters may have been compromised during the surgery. In the absence of cardiac failure or fluid overload, IV Hartmann's solution 500 mL may be used intravenously as the initial fluid challenge while steps are underway to identify the cause for low urine output. If the urine output is satisfactory, the bladder catheter can usually be removed on the first post-operative day once the patient is tolerating oral fluids well and is able to **mobilize** to pass urine on her own. Subsequent ability to void must be assessed to avoid bladder overdistension

4. **Analgesia and ambulation**—for the first 24–48 h, parenteral analgesics or patient-controlled analgesia may be given, together with an antiemetic such as metoclopramide. Thereafter, oral analgesics may suffice. To avoid risk of DVT for low-risk women, early mobilization and hydration are advised. For moderate- and high-risk women, a variety of thromboprophylaxis, such as TED stockings and/or LMWH, is recommended. It is standard practice in most hospitals to administer LMWH (dalteparin 5000 U SC once daily) after C/S until the woman is freely mobile. Deep breathing should also be encouraged to overcome post-operative atelectasis

5. **Routine investigations**—FBC is usually performed on the second or third post-operative day to detect anaemia. Serum electrolytes should be checked in patients on prolonged IV fluid therapy

6. **Wound care**—the incision is usually inspected on the third post-operative day and the sutures or clips removed (if required) on the fifth day for Pfannenstiel incision and on the seventh day for midline incision. If the patient complains of severe incisional pain, the wound should be evaluated for infection or haematoma

7. **Breast care**—breastfeeding should be gently encouraged for all mothers as early as possible and can be initiated soon after the delivery once the mother feels ready

8. **Antibiotics**—only single-dose prophylactic antibiotics are recommended just before the skin incision for Caesarean deliveries. Women with clinical chorioamnionitis need aggressive antibiotic therapy until they are afebrile, have no signs of infection, such as uterine tenderness, and for a further 1 week

9. **Prophylactic oxytocin**—infusion for 4–6 h, following the delivery, to facilitate uterine contraction may be recommended in women who have had overdistended uteri (big baby, twins) or a long labour with inadequate uterine activity

10. **Debriefing**—women who have had a C/S should be offered the opportunity to discuss the reasons for their surgery and implications for future pregnancies.

Possible complications in the post-operative period

- Immediate—haemorrhage, amniotic fluid embolism, Mendelson's syndrome (aspiration pneumonia). Haemorrhage is more likely to be atonic in the early post-operative period (though unidentified trauma at the time of surgery is possible). Later, bleeding is usually associated with endometritis or, less commonly, retained tissue
- Early—atelectasis, chest infection, chorioamnionitis, thrombophlebitis, breast engorgement, urinary retention, UTI, paralytic ileus, pelvic haematoma and abscess, wound infection, wound breakdown, DVT, PE
- Others—breastfeeding problems, post-natal depression/blues/psychosis.
- Late—abdominal adhesions, scar rupture, and placenta praevia/accreta in future pregnancies.

Further reading

Baskett TF, Calder AA, Arulkumaran S (2007). Caesarean section. In *Munro Kerr's operative obstetrics*, 11th edn, pp. 155–66. Elsevier Saunders, London.

National Institute for Health and Clinical Excellence (2011). *Caesarean section.* NICE clinical guideline 132. Available at: <http://www.nice.org.uk/nicemedia/live/13620/57163/57163.pdf>.

Care pathway for immediate post-operative care after Caesarean section

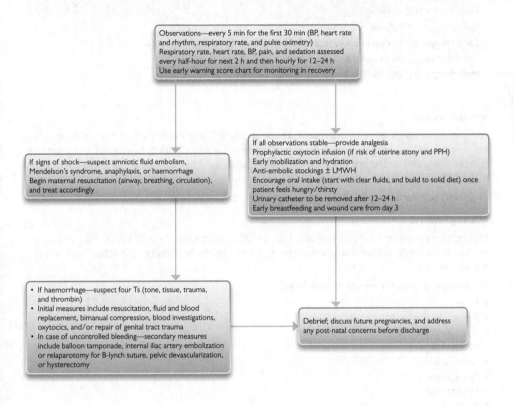

Observations—every 5 min for the first 30 min (BP, heart rate and rhythm, respiratory rate, and pulse oximetry)
Respiratory rate, heart rate, BP, pain, and sedation assessed every half-hour for next 2 h and then hourly for 12–24 h
Use early warning score chart for monitoring in recovery

If signs of shock—suspect amniotic fluid embolism, Mendelson's syndrome, anaphylaxis, or haemorrhage
Begin maternal resuscitation (airway, breathing, circulation), and treat accordingly

If all observations stable—provide analgesia
Prophylactic oxytocin infusion (if risk of uterine atony and PPH)
Early mobilization and hydration
Anti-embolic stockings ± LMWH
Encourage oral intake (start with clear fluids, and build to solid diet) once patient feels hungry/thirsty
Urinary catheter to be removed after 12–24 h
Early breastfeeding and wound care from day 3

- If haemorrhage—suspect four Ts (tone, tissue, trauma, and thrombin)
- Initial measures include resuscitation, fluid and blood replacement, bimanual compression, blood investigations, oxytocics, and/or repair of genital tract trauma
- In case of uncontrolled bleeding—secondary measures include balloon tamponade, internal iliac artery embolization or relaparotomy for B-lynch suture, pelvic devascularization, or hysterectomy

Debrief; discuss future pregnancies, and address any post-natal concerns before discharge

Post-partum pyrexia and puerperal sepsis

Key learning points

Causes are multifactorial

Early recognition is vital in prevention of maternal morbidity and mortality

Consider use of sepsis bundle

Multidisciplinary approach to treatment is mandatory.

Introduction

Post-partum pyrexia is defined as a temperature rise above 38°C, maintained over 24 h or recurring during the period from the end of the first to the end of the tenth day after childbirth or abortion. Endometritis is the most common infection in the post-partum period. Sepsis is defined as infection plus systemic manifestations of infection.

At present, post-partum sepsis is the leading cause of direct maternal death.

Management

Early recognition is essential. Abdominal pain, fever (>38°C), and tachycardia (>90 bpm in the puerperium) are indications for IV antibiotics and senior clinical review. Mastitis, as a source of infection, may be easily overlooked.

Symptoms suggestive of pyrexia and sepsis include:

- Fever
- Rigor
- Foul-smelling lochia
- Abdominal pain
- Tachycardia
- Tachypnoea
- Hypotension
- Erythema
- Oedema
- Tenderness and discharge from the wound or episiotomy site
- Patients with pyelonephritis or UTIs may have costovertebral angle tenderness or suprapubic pain.

Investigations

- Temperature
- BP
- Respiratory rate
- Urine output
- Blood count
- CRP
- Electrolytes
- Blood cultures
- Urinalysis with cultures
- Vaginal swab
- Wound swab
- ABGs
- Serum lactate ≥4 mmol/L is indicative of tissue hypoperfusion
- Pelvic ultrasonography for detecting retained products of conception or pelvic abscess
- CXR is important to rule out pneumonia.

Treatment

Employment of a sepsis bundle within a very short time frame is recommended to save lives. This involves treatment with high-dose antibiotics prior to making a diagnosis. This also involves multidisciplinary involvement, anaesthetic review, aggressive fluid management, and oxygen therapy in the initial period, as post-partum pyrexia can rapidly deteriorate to puerperal sepsis and cardiovascular collapse.

High-dose IV broad-spectrum antibiotic therapy should be started as early as possible. It may be necessary to admit a patient to HDU for cardiac monitoring and support.

Further reading

Centre for Maternal and Child Enquiries (CMACE) (2011). Saving Mothers' Lives: reviewing maternal deaths to make motherhood safer: 2006–08. The Eighth Report on Confidential Enquiries into Maternal Deaths in the United Kingdom. *British Journal of Obstetrics and Gynaecology*, **118** (Suppl 1), 1–203. Available at: <http://onlinelibrary.wiley.com/doi/10.1111/j.1471-0528.2010.02847.x/pdf>.

Cunningham G, Levano KJ, Gilstrap LC, *et al.* (2005). *Williams obstetrics*, 22nd edn. McGraw-Hill Medical, [city].

Royal College of Obstetricians and Gynaecologists (2012). *Bacterial sepsis following pregnancy.* Green-top guideline No. 64b. Available at: <http://www.rcog.org.uk/files/rcog-corp/25.4.12GTG64b.pdf>.

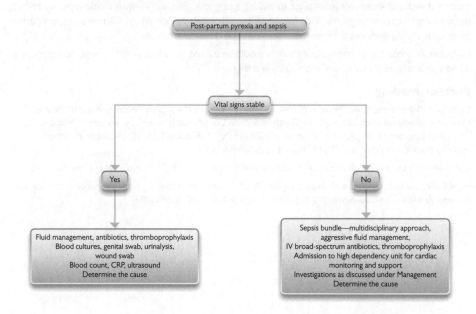

Care pathway for post-partum pyrexia and puerperal sepsis

Post-partum pyrexia and sepsis

Vital signs stable

Yes

No

Fluid management, antibiotics, thromboprophylaxis
Blood cultures, genital swab, urinalysis,
wound swab
Blood count, CRP, ultrasound
Determine the cause

Sepsis bundle—multidisciplinary approach,
aggressive fluid management,
IV broad-spectrum antibiotics, thromboprophylaxis
Admission to high dependency unit for cardiac
monitoring and support
Investigations as discussed under Management
Determine the cause

SECTION 3

Non-urgent gynaecology

Menorrhagia

Menorrhagia

Key learning points

Causes of menorrhagia can be both local and systemic

Most investigations can be delivered in a 'one-stop' setting

Management options increasingly non-surgical or minimally invasive.

Definition

- Excessive menstrual loss which interferes with the woman's physical, emotional, social, and material quality of life
- Also defined as menstrual blood loss >80 mL per period, commonly a subjective assessment.

Epidemiology

- One in four women suffer from menstrual problems over their lifetime, and 6.5% of all women aged 12–51 have heavy menstrual bleeding.

Causes

- Local
  - Fibroids
  - Endometrial polyps
  - Endometrial hyperplasia and carcinoma
- Systemic disorders
  - Thyroid disease
  - Clotting disorders
- Iatrogenic
  - Oral anticoagulants
  - Intrauterine contraceptive devices (IUCDs)
- **Dysfunctional uterine bleeding** (where no local or systemic cause is found).

The most common cause is dysfunctional uterine bleeding.

History

- Nature of bleeding and impact on the quality of life
- Relevant history to rule out systemic and iatrogenic causes
- Associated symptoms such as intermenstrual bleeding, post-coital bleeding, pelvic pain, and pressure symptoms, which indicate a likely pelvic pathology
- Measuring blood loss is not recommended.

Examination

Abdominal and pelvic examination if suspecting local causes.

Investigations

- FBC to exclude anaemia
- TFTs and clotting tests where indicated through clinical suspicion
- Pelvic ultrasound for identifying pelvic pathology, e.g. fibroids, adnexal masses, and endometrial polyps. Indications include an enlarged uterus or pelvic mass on examination or failure of first line of management

- Endometrial biopsy to exclude endometrial cancer or hyperplasia. It is usually indicated in all women over 45, women under 45 if there are suspicious findings on ultrasound, and in cases of first-line treatment failure
- Hysteroscopy is indicated if ultrasound suspects intrauterine pathology, e.g. endometrial polyps, submucous fibroids, and endometrial carcinoma.

Management

- Management should aim to improve the quality of life
- Management will depend on the cause of menorrhagia, desire for fertility, and patient choice.

Medical treatment

- Medical treatment is the first line of management for dysfunctional uterine bleeding or fibroids <3 cm in diameter not distorting the uterine cavity
- It includes hormonal methods like levonorgestrel-releasing intrauterine system (LNG-IUS), combined oral contraceptives, and progestogens (oral or injectables)
- Non-hormonal methods include tranexamic acid and non-steroidal anti-inflammatory drugs (NSAIDs)
- Gonadotrophin-releasing hormone (GnRH) analogue can be used as second-line treatment if primary treatment fails.

Surgical treatment

- Surgical treatment should be usually employed if medical treatment fails
- Endometrial ablation should be used in women with normal uterus, uterine size less than a 10-week pregnancy, uterine fibroids <3 cm in diameter, and who do not wish to conceive
- Hysteroscopic removal of endometrial polyps and submucous fibroids can alleviate symptoms of menorrhagia
- Uterine artery embolization (UAE) and myomectomy should be considered in women with large fibroids (>3 cm) who wish to retain their uterus and potentially their fertility (see Chapter 66 on fibroids)
- Hysterectomy should be considered if other treatment methods have failed and the woman does not wish to retain her uterus and fertility. It should not be used as the first line of treatment.

Further reading

Apgar BS, Kaufman AH, George-Nwogu U, Kittendorf A (2007). Treatment of menorrhagia. *American Family Physician*, **75**, 1813–19.

National Institute for Health and Clinical Excellence (2007). *Heavy menstrual bleeding*. NICE clinical guideline 44. Available at: <http://www.nice.org.uk/nicemedia/pdf/cg44niceguideline.pdf>.

Prentice A (1999). Medical management of menorrhagia. *BMJ*, **319**, 1343–5.

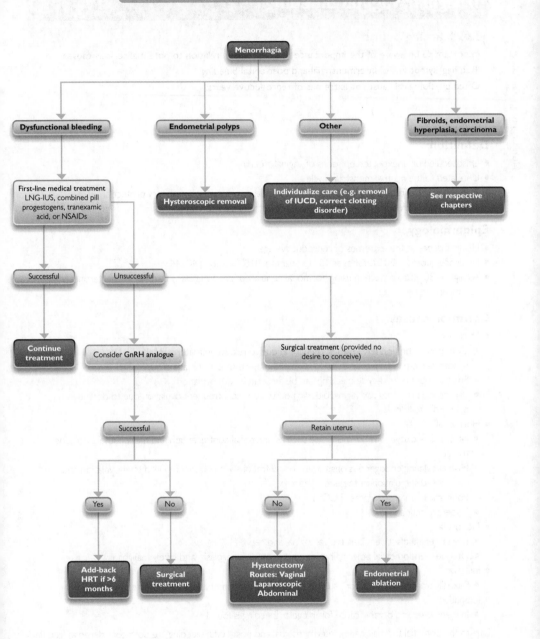

Algorithm for menorrhagia

Menorrhagia

- **Dysfunctional bleeding**
  - **First-line medical treatment** LNG-IUS, combined pill progestogens, tranexamic acid, or NSAIDs
    - Successful
      - **Continue treatment**
    - Unsuccessful
      - Consider GnRH analogue
        - Successful
          - Yes
            - **Add-back HRT if >6 months**
          - No
            - **Surgical treatment**
      - Surgical treatment (provided no desire to conceive)
        - Retain uterus
          - No
            - **Hysterectomy Routes: Vaginal Laparoscopic Abdominal**
          - Yes
            - **Endometrial ablation**
- **Endometrial polyps**
  - **Hysteroscopic removal**
- **Other**
  - **Individualize care (e.g. removal of IUCD, correct clotting disorder)**
- **Fibroids, endometrial hyperplasia, carcinoma**
  - **See respective chapters**

Irregular vaginal bleeding

Key learning points

Important to be aware of the importance of symptoms in relation to potential serious causes

'Red flag' symptoms of intermenstrual and post-coital bleeding

Often physiological causes at extremes of reproductive years.

Definition

- Unscheduled or unexpected episodes of vaginal bleeding
- Unrelated to the normal menstrual cycle
- Bleeding may be frequent, prolonged, heavy, or spotting not requiring sanitary protection
- Irregular vaginal bleeding may also be associated with sexual intercourse.

Epidemiology

- High incidence at the extremes of reproductive age
- Incidence quoted—20.8% for ages 15–19 years to 10.8% for ages 40–44 years
- As high as 30–40% in women using hormonal contraception, particularly users of progesterone-only contraception.

Common causes

- Physiological
  - Common in the first few years of menarche due to relative immaturity of the hypothalamic-pituitary-ovarian axis. Pelvic pathology is rare in this age group
  - Small amount of mid-cycle bleeding can be associated with ovulation
  - Perimenopausal irregular vaginal bleeding occurs due to infrequent ovulation due to decline in primordial follicles
- Hormonal
  - Iatrogenic—exogenous hormone use such as hormonal contraception and menopausal hormone therapy
  - High circulating endogenous oestrogen concentrations with obesity can lead to anovulation and unopposed stimulation of the endometrium
  - Polycystic ovarian syndrome (PCOS)
  - Hyperprolactinaemia
- Neoplasia
  - Lower genital tract neoplasia (vulva, vagina, and cervix)
  - Uterine—endometrial polyps, fibroids, endometrial hyperplasia, and rarely malignancy
- Infective
  - Sexually transmitted infections such as Chlamydia, Trichomonas, and viral warts
- Idiopathic
  - In many cases, no organic cause for irregular bleeding is found.

Due to the potential for malignancy, intermenstrual and post-coital bleeding are both considered as 'red flag' symptoms, worthy of more urgent investigation.

Clinical assessment

- Usually generally well but may suffer from a poor quality of life
- May be anaemic, especially if there has been a delay in presentation
- Anaemia is normally of gradual progression—patients are haemodynamically stable

- The relationship of any irregular bleeding to the menarche, menopause, or the current menstrual cycle should be documented
- History of past and present exogenous hormone use must be elicited
- History of post-coital bleeding may suggest underlying neoplastic lesions of the lower genital tract.

Examination should include:

- BMI
- Signs of hyperandrogenism (acanthosis nigricans, hirsutism, and acne)
- Examination of the abdomen and pelvis should include visualization of the lower genital tract.

Investigations

Investigations are generally few and refined, according to clinical presentation.

- FBC
- Genital swabs to exclude STI
- Serum hormonal assessments for suspected endocrine abnormalities
- Pelvic ultrasound to exclude pelvic pathology. Its diagnostic accuracy is limited due to high sensitivity but low specificity
- A negative ultrasound is highly reassuring to the patient
- Hysteroscopy is not routinely indicated, unless ultrasound demonstrates suspected pathology.

Management

In idiopathic cases of irregular bleeding, the first line of treatment is usually:

- Hormonal manipulation to regulate the cycles. Combined oral contraceptive pill (COCP) or progestogens are helpful to restore cycle regularity and control heavy bleeding
- Submucous fibroids or endometrial polyps, detected by USS, can be removed, using modern hysteroscopic techniques.

Most women require reassurance, as this is normally a self-limiting condition.

Common pitfalls

Pregnancy should always be excluded by performing a urinary pregnancy test to rule out pregnancy-related bleeding.

Further reading

Faculty of Sexual and Reproductive Healthcare Clinical Effectiveness Unit, in collaboration with the Royal College of Obstetricians and Gynaecologists (2009). *Management of unscheduled bleeding in women using hormonal contraception*. FSHR guidance. Available at: <http://www.rcog.org.uk/files/rcog-corp/UnscheduledBleeding23092009.pdf>.

Munster K, Schmidt L, Helm P (1992). Length and variation in the menstrual cycle—a cross-sectional study from a Danish county. *British Journal of Obstetrics and Gynaecology*, **99**, 422–9.

National Collaborating Centre for Women's and Children's Health (2007). *Heavy menstrual bleeding*. Clinical guideline. Available from: <http://www.nice.org.uk/nicemedia/live/11002/30401/30401.pdf>.

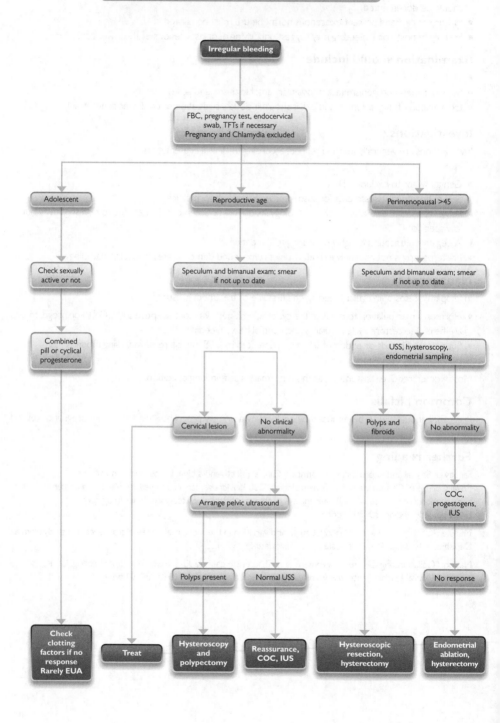

Algorithm for irregular vaginal bleeding

Irregular bleeding

FBC, pregnancy test, endocervical
swab, TFTs if necessary
Pregnancy and Chlamydia excluded

Adolescent

Check sexually
active or not

Combined
pill or cyclical
progesterone

Check
clotting
factors if no
response
Rarely EUA

Reproductive age

Speculum and bimanual exam; smear
if not up to date

Cervical lesion

No clinical
abnormality

Arrange pelvic ultrasound

Polyps present

Normal USS

Treat

Hysteroscopy
and
polypectomy

Reassurance,
COC, IUS

Perimenopausal >45

Speculum and bimanual exam; smear
if not up to date

USS, hysteroscopy,
endometrial sampling

Polyps and
fibroids

No abnormality

COC,
progestogens,
IUS

No response

Hysteroscopic
resection,
hysterectomy

Endometrial
ablation,
hysterectomy

Amenorrhoea

Key learning points

Investigations for primary amenorrhoea should be undertaken earlier in the absence of other features of puberty

Hypothalamic causes are common in both primary and secondary amenorrhoea

Pregnancy is the commonest cause of secondary amenorrhoea and should be excluded prior to investigation

Psychological counselling is important in the management of patients with ovarian failure, Müllerian structural abnormalities, and intersex conditions.

Definition

Primary amenorrhoea

- Absence of menses by 15 years in the presence of normal growth and secondary sexual characteristics. However, evaluations should commence earlier (by age 13) if the pubertal growth spurt and secondary sexual characteristics are absent.

Secondary amenorrhoea

- The absence of menses for 6 or more months in a woman who had menses previously.

Causes

The causes of primary and secondary amenorrhoea are shown in Table 1.

Assessment and management

Primary amenorrhoea

History

- Seek other stages of puberty
  - Growth spurt, axillary and pubic hair, breast development
    - Lack of pubertal development suggests an ovarian/pituitary failure or a chromosomal abnormality
  - A family history of delayed or absent puberty
  - Any neonatal and childhood diseases
    - Neonatal crisis, suggestive of adrenal and chronic disease, can cause hypothalamic-pituitary dysfunction
  - Recent changes in weight, exercise habits, or recent life events causing stress
  - Drug history, e.g. use of metoclopramide, antipsychotics
  - Symptoms of genital tract obstruction such as cyclical abdominal pain.

Examination

- Height, weight, arm span, pubertal development
- Breast development
- Genital examination
  - Clitoral size, pubertal hair development
  - Presence of cervix and uterus (by rectal examination if vaginal examination not possible)
- Hirsutism, acne, striae, increased pigmentation
- Vitiligo—may be seen associated with autoimmune conditions of ovarian failure
- Features of Turner's syndrome—low hairline, webbed neck, widely spaced nipples.

Investigations

- Pelvic ultrasound

Table 1 Causes of primary and secondary amenorrhoea

Primary amenorrhoea	Secondary amenorrhoea
Constitutional delay	Pregnancy
Hypothalamic causes	Hypothalamic dysfunction
Functional	Functional
Secondary to eating disorders, exercise, or stress	Secondary to eating disorders, exercise, and stress
Congenital GnRH deficiency including Kallmann's syndrome (associated with anosmia)	Nutritional deficiencies, systemic illness
Pituitary causes	Pituitary disease
Prolactinoma	Hyperprolactinaemia
Cranial tumours	Other sellar masses
Gonadal	Thyroid disease
Gonadal agenesis—Turner's syndrome (45,XO), partial deletions, and structural derangements	Hypothyroidism
Müllerian agenesis	Hyperthyroidism
Mayer–Rokitansky–Küster–Hauser syndrome	Ovarian causes
Outflow obstruction	PCOS
Imperforate hymen	Premature ovarian failure
Transverse vaginal septum	Uterine causes
Intersex	Asherman syndrome
Complete androgen insensitivity	
5-alpha reductase deficiency in 46XY	
17-alpha hydroxylase deficiency	
Absent testis determining factor (Ullrich–Turner syndrome)	

- • Assess the presence of cervix, uterus, and ovaries
- • For haematocolpos or haematometra
- Serum FSH, testosterone, and prolactin
- Karyotype.

Treatment

Aims of treatment:

- Correcting underlying pathology, if possible
- Achieve fertility
- Prevention of complications of the disease (bone loss).

Main treatment interventions:

- Lifestyle modifications and other behavioural therapy in functional hypothalamic amenorrhoea
- Surgery
  - • Corrective for anatomical lesions
  - • Gonadectomy in Y chromosome conditions. This may be delayed until after puberty in complete androgen insensitivity syndrome to facilitate normal growth spurt and feminization. Tumours do not develop until after this time
- Hormone replacement therapy (HRT) in premature ovarian failure
- PCOS is a rare cause of primary amenorrhoea
  - • Treatment is aimed at achieving desired goals
    - ○ Contraceptive pills to regularize the menses
    - ○ Ovulation induction to improve fertility
    - ○ Withdrawal bleeds to reduce risk of endometrial hyperplasia
  - • Fertility treatment, depending on the abnormality
    - ○ Behavioural therapy and specific treatments for hypothalamic-pituitary causes
    - ○ Oocyte donation for ovarian failure and gonadal dysgenesis
    - ○ Surrogacy in the absence of uterus
  - • Psychological counselling is also required in ovarian failure, absent Müllerian structures, or in intersex conditions.

Secondary amenorrhoea

- First, rule out pregnancy.

History

- Recent changes in weight, diet, or physical exercise
- Chronic medical illness
- Drug history
  - Recent use of oral contraceptive pill, danazol, or high-dose progestogens
  - Other medications, e.g. metoclopramide, antipsychotics, etc.
- Symptoms of hypothalamic-pituitary disease
  - Headache, visual field defects, fatigue, polyuria, or polydipsia
- Look for symptoms of oestrogen deficiency
  - Hot flushes, vaginal dryness, poor sleep, decreased libido
- Elicit any history of endometrial injury
  - Dilatation and curettage, uterine infections.

Examination

- BMI—obesity as well as low BMI
- Evidence of thyroid disease, e.g. goitre, tachycardia, tremors
- Features of PCOS, e.g. hirsutism, acne, striae, acanthosis nigricans
- Breast examination for galactorrhoea
- Genital examination for evidence of oestrogen deficiency.

Investigations

- Basic endocrinological assessment
  - Serum FSH—for ovarian failure and pituitary underactivity
  - TSH for thyroid disease
  - Prolactin for pituitary adenoma
- Androgen levels and free androgen index (FAI)
  - Androgen levels can be normal in PCOS, and, therefore, FAI should be assessed

$$FAI = (total\ testosterone \times 100) / SHBG$$

- Pituitary MRI for any pituitary tumours
- Hysteroscopy to assess the endometrium.

Treatment

Hypothalamic amenorrhoea
  - Lifestyle changes, cognitive behavioural therapy

Hyperprolactinaemia
  - Microadenomas—dopamine agonists such as bromocriptine and cabergoline
  - Macroadenomas—may require surgery

Premature ovarian failure
  - Oestrogen therapy to prevent bone loss
  - Combined contraceptive pill or hormone replacement therapy

PCOS
  - Depending on the woman's desires
    - Contraceptive pills to regularize the menses
    - Ovulation induction to restore fertility
    - Progestogen induced withdrawal bleeds to reduce the risk of endometrial hyperplasia

Further reading

Dickerson EH, Raghunath AS, Atkin SL (2009). Rational testing: initial investigation of amenorrhoea. *BMJ*, **339**, 455–7

Practice Committee of the American Society for Reproductive Medicine (2008). Current evaluation of amenorrhea. *Fertility and Sterility*, **90** (Suppl 3), S219–25.

Welt CK and Barbieri RL (2013). *Etiology, diagnosis, and treatment of primary amenorrhea.* Available at: <http://www.uptodate.com/contents/etiology-diagnosis-and-treatment-of-primary-amenorrhea>.

Algorithm for amenorrhoea

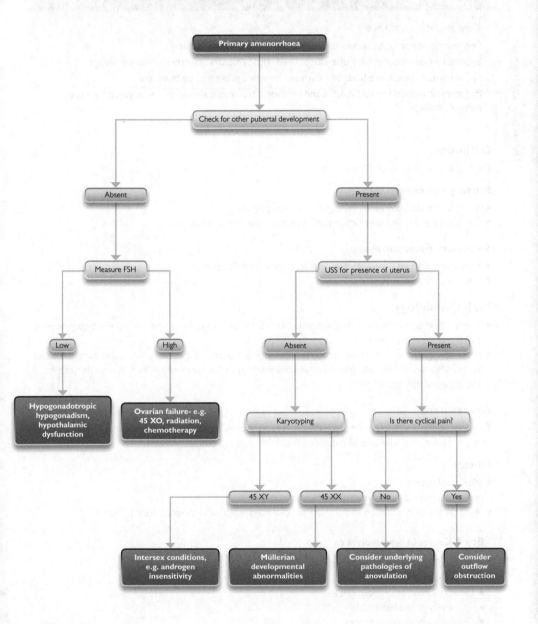

Dysmenorrhoea

Key learning points

Primary dysmenorrhoea occurs in the first few years of menstruation

Secondary dysmenorrhoea is often associated with symptoms of other pelvic pathology

Non-pharmacological methods of treatment have not proved to be beneficial

Patients not responding to NSAIDs and hormonal treatment should be investigated for other pelvic pathology.

Definition

Defined as difficult or painful menstruation.

Primary dysmenorrhoea

- Symptoms in the absence of any significant pelvic pathology
- Occurs in the first few years after menarche and is spasmodic in nature.

Secondary dysmenorrhoea

- Symptoms resulting from anatomic or macroscopic pelvic pathology
- Generally congestive in nature.

Pathophysiology

- Primary dysmenorrhoea—by myometrial ischaemia due to frequent and prolonged uterine contractions and is prostaglandin-mediated
- Secondary dysmenorrhoea often precedes the menses and may be associated with other symptoms such as dyspareunia and dyschezia (painful bowel movements). In the presence of fibroids, it is often due to the increased menstrual flow.

Assessment

Diagnosis of primary dysmenorrhoea is clinical. A history of dysmenorrhoea in the absence of any symptoms or signs suggestive of a pelvic pathology. See Box 1 for causes of dysmenorrhoea.

History

- Menstrual history
  - Age at menarche and onset of dysmenorrhoea
  - Cycle regularity, duration and amount of flow, intermenstrual or premenstrual bleeding

---

Box 1 Causes of dysmenorrhoea

- PG-mediated primary dysmenorrhoea
- Endometriosis
- Pelvic inflammatory disease (PID)
- Ovarian cysts and tumours
- Cervical stenosis or occlusions
- Adenomyosis
- Fibroids
- Uterine polyps
- Intrauterine adhesions
- Intrauterine contraceptive device
- Pelvic congestion syndrome.

- Features of the pain
  - The onset in relation to flow and severity
  - Nature and location of pain
  - Any association with nausea, vomiting, diarrhoea, back pain, or headache
- Response to medication
  - Type of medications used so far and symptom improvement with these
- Effect of the symptoms on daily activities and sexual function.

Examination

- Abdominal examination
  - Lower abdominal tenderness
- Vaginal and bimanual examination
  - Size, mobility, and tenderness of the uterus
  - Evidence of pelvic pathology in the adnexae
  - Uterosacral ligaments thickened and nodular, with focal tenderness.

Investigations

- Genital swabs for infection, including Chlamydia and gonorrhoea
- Pelvic USS
  - May aid in diagnosis of pelvic pathologies such as fibroids, adenomyosis, endometriosis
- Diagnostic laparoscopy
  - Gold standard in diagnosis of endometriosis
  - Also useful in diagnosis of pelvic adhesions and chronic PID.

Treatment

Primary dysmenorrhoea

Non-pharmacological methods

- Dietary modifications, vitamins, herbal therapies, and physical exercise have been proposed. However, the supporting evidence is not strong enough, to date, to recommend these in routine clinical practice.

Pharmacological methods

- Cyclo-oxygenase (COX) inhibitors
  - Since the pain is PG-mediated, COX inhibitors are effective in improving symptoms. The treatment success rate could be as high as 70–90%
  - The effects are brought about by the reduction of PG in the menstrual blood as well as by reducing the amount of flow
  - The treatment should be commenced 1–2 days prior to menses and continued for duration of the pain
  - Effective NSAIDs include ibuprofen, naproxen, ketoprofen, and mefenamic acid.
  - COX-2 inhibitors are more potent PG inhibitors. However, the higher cost and potential risks have limited their use
- Hormonal treatment
  - COCP is preferred in those who do not wish for fertility and those who do not respond to, or tolerate, NSAIDs
  - All regimes of COCP are effective. Symptom improvement has been seen with levonorgestrel IUS (Mirena®) and etonogestrel implants (Implanon®) as well
  - If a patient is resistant to treatment, further evaluation should be carried out to exclude any pelvic pathology, such as endometriosis, causing secondary dysmenorrhoea
  - Treatment of secondary dysmenorrhoea is mainly by treating the underlying pathology, though treatment modalities may give some symptomatic relief.

Further reading

Calis KA (2013). *Dysmenorrhea*. Available at: <http://emedicine.medscape.com/article/253812-overview>.

Smith RP and Kaunitz AM (2013). *Treatment of primary dysmenorrhea in adult women*. Available at: <http://www.uptodate.com/contents/treatment-of-primary-dysmenorrhea-in-adult-women>.

Society of Gynaecologists of Canada (2005). *Primary dysmenorrhea consensus guideline*. SOGC clinical practice guideline No. 169. Available at: <http://sogc.org/wp-content/uploads/2013/01/169E-CPG-December2005.pdf>.

Algorithm for dysmenorrhoea

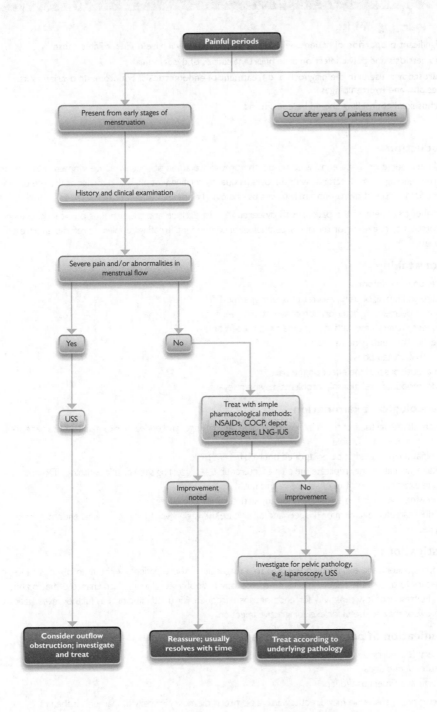

Painful intercourse

Key learning points

A significant proportion of patients with painful intercourse will have no identifiable cause

Endometriosis and pelvic infection are important causes of dyspareunia

Laparoscopy is useful in the diagnosis and treatment of endometriosis, symptomatic ovarian cysts, adhesions, and hydrosalpinges

Psychosexual counselling should be considered.

Introduction

Painful intercourse or dyspareunia is common; the prevalence amongst sexually active women is as high as 46%. The aetiology is multifactorial, with the pain frequently relating to a physical disorder at the site of tenderness. Some cases of dyspareunia may have a psychological element.

The goal of treatment of the patient with dyspareunia is to exclude and treat serious physical disease and then correct any coexisting or remaining psychological component. Treating couples is preferable to treating individuals.

History taking

- Duration of symptoms
- Nature and timing of pain (visceral, muscular, spasmodic)
- Any improvement or deterioration of symptoms over time
- Frequency (every time with intercourse or at specific times)
- Superficial or deep penetration
- Masturbation, tampons
- Sexual positions and the effect on the pain
- Libido, mood, and relationship problems may be relevant.

Gynaecological examination

- Be considerate to the fact this may be a psychological challenge, and endeavour to maintain the patient's comfort as much as possible
- Examination may need to be postponed until a different clinic visit
- Digital examination may replicate the pain of intercourse—suggesting site-specific pathology. Do not pursue examination in cases of severe vaginismus
- Inspect the vulva and hymen carefully for any structural abnormalities
- Conduct targeted examination. Inspect and/or palpate the vaginal vault for rectovaginal endometriotic nodules.

Investigations

Commonly, history and examination will lead to a diagnosis. In those patients without an obvious cause, it is necessary to discuss the relative merits of laparoscopy (risk of visceral injury, high chance of finding nothing) and ultrasound (low sensitivity for endometriosis, frequent incidental findings) as further investigations. Genital swabs may be useful for excluding active infection.

Classification of painful intercourse

- Primary/secondary
- Persistent/conditional
- Superficial or insertional/deep.

Characterizing dyspareunia may direct towards a particular diagnosis. Primary dyspareunia is the first presentation where intercourse has either only just commenced and is painful or has always been painful. Secondary dyspareunia is the onset of painful sex in someone who has previously not experienced it.

Causes of painful intercourse

Common physical causes of painful intercourse may be classified by reproductive stage. Some conditions span all of the reproductive life.

- All women
  - Vaginismus
  - IBS (including chronic constipation)
  - Inflammatory bowel disease
  - Cystitis
  - Vulvodynia
  - Vaginal dryness
- All women of reproductive age
  - Endometriosis
  - Chronic PID
  - Pelvic mass
    - Fibroids
    - Ovarian cysts
- Nulliparous women
  - Imperforate hymen, vaginal septum
- Parous women
  - Perineal trauma—scar tissue formation
  - Prolapse
- Peri- or post-menopausal women
  - Atrophic vaginitis
  - Diverticular disease
  - Lichen sclerosis.

Management

General advice

All patients with dyspareunia may benefit from simple advice, which they may have already exhausted through trial and error or in consultation with their general practitioner (GP). Lubrication, short-course topical oestrogen, different sexual positions, or non-penetrative sexual activity may be all that is required to provide symptomatic relief.

Management of specific conditions

If a clear cause has been identified, such as endometriosis, then treatment should be directed towards management of the diagnosis. This could include surgery for a specific indication.

Vulval conditions may respond to topical treatment with steroids, emollients, or antifungals. Consider a tertiary referral or biopsy.

Initial empirical management for endometriosis by oral progestogens, IUS, or COCP on a continuous basis or with GnRh agonists can be instigated prior to a formal diagnosis by laparoscopy, as even those patients without endometriosis may improve. Up to 60% of cases of endometriosis are missed at laparoscopy.

Chronic pelvic pain with dyspareunia

Consider referral to a specialist or tertiary centre. IBS-type symptoms may be alleviated by a high-fibre or low-residue diet. Nerve entrapment pain may be responsive to local anaesthetic injection (by a pain specialist). Pain on movement may respond to physiotherapy.

If pain is predominantly cyclical, a trial of ovarian suppression, with combined oral contraceptive or GnRH agonists, with or without HRT, may be appropriate.

Further reading

Royal College of Obstetricians and Gynaecologists (2006). *The investigation and management of endometriosis.* Green-top guideline No. 24. Available at: <http://www.rcog.org.uk/womens-health/clinical-guidance/investigation-and-management-endometriosis-green-top-24>.

Royal College of Obstetricians and Gynaecologists (2012). *The initial management of chronic pelvic pain.* Green-top guideline No. 41. Available at: <http://www.rcog.org.uk/womens-health/clinical-guidance/initial-management-chronic-pelvic-pain-green-top-41>.

Abnormal cervical smears

Key learning points

The traditional cervical smear has recently been replaced by liquid-based cytology that can also detect human papillomavirus (HPV)

Over 93% of smears are negative

'See and treat' colposcopy care pathways are appropriate in cases of suspected high-grade lesions

Follow-up with a 'test of cure' protocol reduces the frequency of follow-up visits.

Introduction

In England, women between the ages of 25 and 64 years are invited to attend for cervical screening. The frequency of screening intervals is every 3 years for women aged 25–49 years and every 5 years for women between the ages of 50 and 64 years.

Cervical cytological screening aims to identify dyskaryotic cells arising from the transformation zone of the cervix. The conventional Papanicolaou method has recently been replaced by liquid-based cytology that has the advantage of using the same specimen for cytological and HPV testing.

High-risk HPV can be detected in 99.7% of cases of cervical cancer. The most common oncogenic subtypes found in women with cervical carcinoma include HPV 16, 18, 31, 33, 45, and 59.

Epidemiology

Over 4.3 million women were invited in 2010–11 for cervical cytology screening in England, generating under 3.7 million tests. Of the samples tested, 2.8% did not contain adequate material for analysis; 93.4% were negative, and 6.6% were abnormal (borderline 3.5%, mild 1.9%, moderate 0.5%, and severe dyskaryosis 0.6%).

Cervical cytology

Women should be referred to colposcopy clinic if:

- Cytology result of suspicion of invasive cancer or glandular neoplasia
- Moderate or severe dyskaryosis
- Any endocervical cell changes
- Three consecutive inadequate samples
- Three abnormal test results in a 10-year period.

According to the HPV Triage protocol currently being implemented, women with a cytology result showing borderline or mild dyskaryosis will have high-risk HPV testing performed. If high-risk HPV is detected, women are referred to colposcopy clinic. If high-risk HPV testing is negative, women will return to routine screening.

Management

The aim of colposcopic examination is to diagnose precancerous (cervical intraepithelial neoplasia, CIN) or cancerous lesions that may be treated at an early stage. Acetic acid solution (3–5%) or Lugol's iodine are used to improve the visualization of abnormal areas. In order to improve detection of CIN, biopsies can be obtained from the most abnormal appearing area of the cervical epithelium.

If cytological result and colposcopic examination are suggestive of low-grade lesion (CIN1) or CIN1 is confirmed on cervical biopsy, then expectant management, rather than treatment, is recommended. The majority of these lesions regress spontaneously, and only a small percentage progress to high-grade lesions (CIN2/3) or invasive cancer.

Treatment at the first visit (see-and-treat policy) is performed if the cytological result and colposcopic examination are suggestive of high-grade lesions (CIN2/3). Regression rates of CIN2/3 lesions are lower than for CIN1, and, if untreated, these lesions are more likely to progress to invasive carcinoma. Ablative and excisional treatment methods have equally effective cure rates. Excisional methods available include large loop excision of the transformation zone (LLETZ), cold knife, and laser conization. Excisional methods have the advantage of tissue available for histology.

Complications of LLETZ treatment include vaginal bleeding, infection, and cervical stenosis. Controversy still exists with regard to the impact of LLETZ treatment on the risk of preterm delivery.

Follow-up

The 'test of cure' is a new approach that involves a combination of cervical cytology and high-risk HPV testing, following treatment for CIN. It is commonly performed 5–6 months following treatment. High-risk HPV testing is performed for women found to have negative cytology result, or borderline or mild dyskaryosis 6 months following treatment. If high-risk HPV is detected, then colposcopic examination is performed. If high-risk HPV testing is negative, then women return to routine screening.

Until recently, surveillance for women treated for CIN involved annual cytology for up to 10 years following treatment. Implementation of the 'test of cure' protocol reduces the frequency of follow-up visits and appears to be cost-effective.

Further reading

NHS Cancer Screening Programmes (2010). *Colposcopy and programme management*. Guidelines for the NHS Cervical Screening Programme (2nd edn). NHSCSP Publication No. 20. Available at: <http://www.cancerscreening. nhs.uk/cervical/publications/nhscsp20.pdf>.

Noehr B, Jensen A, Frederiksen K, Tabor A, Kjaer SK (2009). Loop electrosurgical excision of the cervix and subsequent risk for spontaneous preterm delivery: a population-based study of singleton deliveries during a 9-year period. *American Journal of Obstetrics & Gynecology*, **201**, 33.e1–6.

The NHS Information Centre, Screening and Immunisations team (2011). *Cervical screening programme, England 2010–11*. The Information Centre for health and social care. Available at: <http://www.cancerscreening.nhs.uk/ cervical/cervical-statistics-bulletin-2010-11.pdf>.

Walboomers JM, Jacobs MV, Manos MM, et al. (1999). Human papillomavirus is a necessary cause of invasive cervical cancer worldwide. *Journal of Pathology*, **189**, 12–19.

Algorithm for HPV triage and test of cure protocol

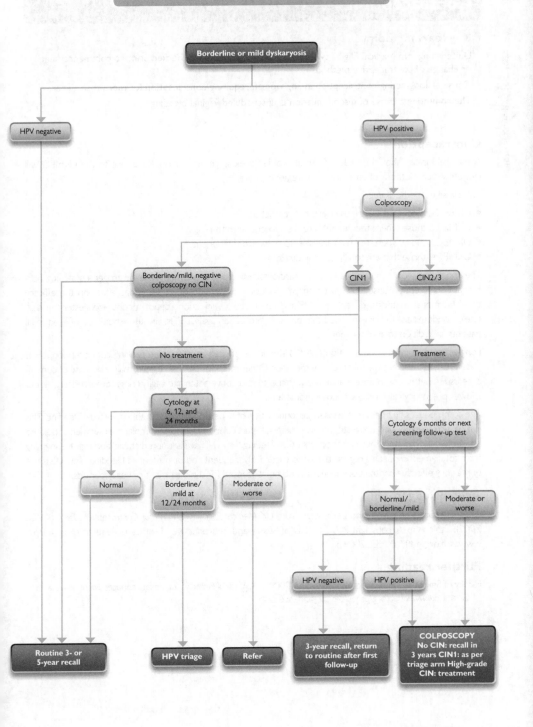

Contraception

Key learning points

United Kingdom Medical Eligibility Criteria (UKMEC) should be checked prior to commencement or change of contraceptive methods

Consider long-acting contraception in any woman requiring contraception for more than a year

The commonest cause of discontinuation is unscheduled vaginal bleeding.

Contraception

A medical history should be taken from all women seeking contraception. Reference to the UKMEC will indicate which methods of contraception are appropriate.

This classifies methods into:

- UKMEC1, those that can be used without restriction
- UKMEC2, those where the benefits are likely to outweigh the risks
- UKMEC3, those where the risks are likely to outweigh the benefits
- UKMEC4, those that are totally contraindicated.

The most common contraindications are cardiovascular risk factors that make oestrogen-containing hormonal contraception unsuitable. Liver enzyme-inducing medication has a significant effect on the efficacy of all hormonal methods, except the IUS and contraceptive injection (depot medroxyprogesterone acetate). Condoms are the only method that provides protection against STIs, and they should be offered to all patients, in addition to another method.

Long-acting reversible contraception (LARC) should be offered to all women seeking contraception for at least a year, as these are the most reliable methods. Other methods are less reliable, mainly because of compliance issues. Better compliance is achieved with the contraceptive patch and vaginal ring, compared to pills, but a lower pregnancy rate has not been demonstrated.

The commonest side effect that leads to discontinuation of a method is unacceptable menstrual bleeding. This is a particular issue with progestogen-only methods, particularly pills and the implant; all women should be advised when they start these methods that the bleeding they will have is 'unpredictable' and may be anything from total amenorrhoea to regular bleeds to excessively frequent and/or prolonged bleeding. The IUS is not only a very effective contraceptive, but has also been licensed for the treatment of heavy periods.

Acknowledgement

UKMEC reproduced with kind permission from *UK Medical Eligibility Criteria for Contraceptive Use (UKMEC 2009)*, Table A, p. 6, copyright 2006, Faculty of Sexual and Reproductive Healthcare. Accessible at: <http://www.fsrh.org/pdfs/UKMEC2009.pdf>

Further reading

Faculty of Sexual and Reproductive Healthcare (2009). *UK Medical Eligibilty Criteria for contraceptive use.* Available at: <http://www.fsrh.org/pages/clinical_guidance.asp>.

Key information for contraception

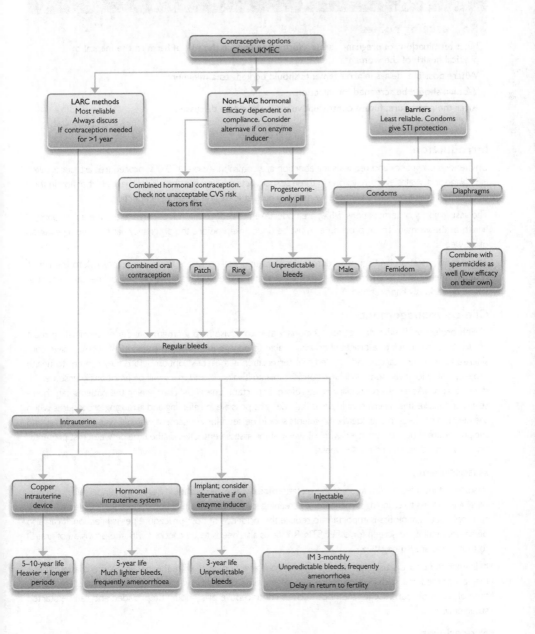

Unwanted pregnancy

Key learning points

Most terminations of pregnancy are performed to reduce the risk of harm to the mental or physical health of the woman

Where possible, delays in arrangements should be kept to a minimum

Women should be screened for infection

After the procedure, future contraceptive plans should be discussed.

Introduction

Unintended pregnancy and requests for abortion are common. About 190 000 procedures are undertaken in England and Wales every year; one in three sexually active women in the UK will have an abortion in their lifetime, and about one-third of these women will have at least one subsequent abortion.

The vast majority of terminations (98%) are undertaken to reduce the risk of harm to the mental or physical health of the woman. These procedures must be undertaken before the pregnancy has reached a gestation of 24 weeks.

There is no gestation limit on procedures which are undertaken where there is a severe risk to the life or health of the mother or where there is substantial risk that the child may have physical or mental abnormalities to be seriously handicapped.

Clinical management

Health professionals who do not feel personally able to advise/help women considering termination must ensure that they refer to a practitioner who is able to engage in a timely manner. Most women have considered their circumstances and decided that termination is their best option before they present to health professionals. However, some will have considerable ambivalence, and many will be emotionally unsettled by their situation. Access to counselling is, therefore, important, unless clinicians seeing the patients can themselves undertake this. There should be as little delay as possible in referring and arranging procedures when the decision has been made. Ideally, all patients should be seen for assessment within 1 week of referral, and the procedure should be arranged within 1 week of the assessment. Overall, the time between first presentation and procedure should be <3 weeks.

Assessment

Assessment includes confirmation of the gestation; ideally, all patients should have a scan undertaken, but certainly easy access to scanning is mandatory. Screening for genital tract infections, particularly Chlamydia, and/or prophylactic antibiotics is important to reduce the incidence of post-procedure pelvic infection. It can also be an opportunity to screen for other STIs. Rh status also needs to be checked with the provision of anti-D to those who are Rh-negative.

It is important to discuss and make a future contraception plan with the patient. Where appropriate, long-acting methods, such as intrauterine devices, implants, or injections, should be fitted/administered at the time of the procedure. Other methods, such as contraceptive pills, should be provided and can be started straightaway.

Procedures

Medical procedures can be undertaken at any gestation. It is a two-stage procedure, with mifepristone given 24–72 h before the administration of a prostaglandin. In pregnancies before 8–9 weeks' gestation, the patient (if appropriate) may be sent home after the administration of the prostaglandin to complete the procedure in their own premises. At later gestations, several doses of prostaglandin may be required, and early discharge is not appropriate.

In very early pregnancy, it is important to exclude an ectopic pregnancy, either before (scan showing an intrauterine yolk sac and/or fetal echo) or after the procedure (by sending products for histology or checking the pregnancy has terminated, with post-procedure β-hCG measurement).

Surgical procedures are not usually undertaken before 7 weeks' gestation. After 12–14 weeks, surgical procedures are much more specialized and should only be undertaken in centres that have developed this expertise.

Follow-up

Follow-up should be discussed and organized with the patient. Routine follow-up has high rates of non-attendance; it is important when there needs to be confirmation that the patient is no longer pregnant, and it is a useful opportunity to encourage the use of effective contraception.

Further reading

Department of Health (2010). *Abortion statistics, England and Wales: 2009*. Statistical Bulletin 2010/1. Available at: <https://www.gov.uk/government/uploads/system/uploads/attachment_data/file/216085/dh_116336.pdf>.

Royal College of Obstetricians and Gynaecologists (2011). *The care of women requesting induced abortion*. Available at: <http://www.rcog.org.uk/guidelines>.

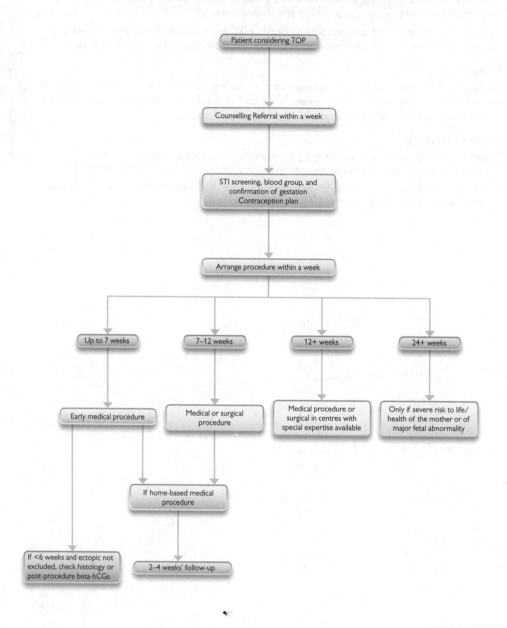

Care pathway for unwanted pregnancy

Patient considering TOP

Counselling Referral within a week

STI screening, blood group, and confirmation of gestation Contraception plan

Arrange procedure within a week

| Up to 7 weeks | 7–12 weeks | 12+ weeks | 24+ weeks |

Early medical procedure

Medical or surgical procedure

Medical procedure or surgical in centres with special expertise available

Only if severe risk to life/ health of the mother or of major fetal abnormality

If home-based medical procedure

If <6 weeks and ectopic not excluded, check histology or post-procedure beta-hCGs

2–4 weeks' follow-up

Recurrent miscarriage

Key learning points

Recurrent miscarriage affects 1% of couples

Its incidence increases with maternal and paternal age

A significant proportion of cases remain unexplained

In unexplained cases, a successful future pregnancy occurs in the region of 75%.

Definition

Miscarriage is defined as the spontaneous loss of a pregnancy before the fetus reaches viability, considered as 24 completed weeks of gestation. Recurrent miscarriage is defined as the loss of three or more consecutive pregnancies. Miscarriage affects 1% of couples trying to conceive.

Epidemiological factors

- Maternal age:
  - Advanced maternal age declines both the number and quality of oocytes (see Table 1)
- Paternal age:
  - Advanced paternal age is also a risk factor for miscarriage
- Previous obstetric history—independent predictor of future pregnancy outcome. The risk of a subsequent miscarriage increases after every successive pregnancy loss:
  - 20% after one miscarriage
  - 30% after two consecutive miscarriages
  - 40% after three consecutive miscarriages
- Obesity—risk of sporadic and recurrent miscarriage is increased.

Aetiology

- Antiphospholipid syndrome (APS) is the association between antiphospholipid antibodies (lupus anticoagulant, anticardiolipin antibodies, and anti-B2 glycoprotein antibodies) and adverse pregnancy outcome or vascular thrombosis. Adverse pregnancy outcomes of APS include recurrent miscarriages, preterm births, and SGA babies. Antiphospholipid antibodies are present in 15% of women with recurrent miscarriage, as opposed to 2% in women with low-risk obstetric history. Without treatment, only 10% of pregnancies in women with recurrent miscarriage and APS will be live born. Antiphospholipid antibodies inhibit the trophoblastic differentiation, cause inflammatory response, and, in later pregnancy, cause thrombosis in the placental vasculature. These effects are reversed by heparin
- Inherited thrombophilic defects (factor V Leiden mutation, prothrombin gene mutation, protein S deficiency) can lead to recurrent miscarriage by causing thrombosis in the uteroplacental vasculature
- PCOS—the risk of recurrent miscarriage is attributed to insulin resistance, hyperinsulinaemia, and hyperandrogenism

Table 1 Risk of miscarriage with maternal age

Maternal age (years)	Risk of miscarriage (%)
12–29	11–13
30–34	15
35–39	25
40–44	51
45 and above	93

- Parental chromosomal rearrangements—balanced chromosomal translocations are present in either partner in 2–5% of recurrent miscarriages. The risk of miscarriage depends on the size of genetic material in the relocated segment
- Embryonic chromosomal abnormalities—increases with maternal age. In couples with recurrent miscarriage, chromosomal abnormalities of the fetus account for 30–60% of further miscarriages
- Uterine malformations—usually coincidental, rather than the cause. Present in 2% of women with normal reproductive history. Prevalence higher in women with second-trimester miscarriage
- Cervical weakness—exact incidence unknown but is a recognized cause of second-trimester miscarriage. Diagnosis is based on clinical history of second-trimester miscarriage, preceded by SROM or painless cervical dilatation
- Immunological conditions, other than APS, as causes of recurrent miscarriage are controversial and not yet proven
- Infection—there is no evidence that TORCH (toxoplasmosis, rubella, cytomegalovirus, hepatitis) infections cause recurrent miscarriage.

Management

Women with recurrent miscarriage should be looked after by a health professional with the necessary skills and expertise. Where available, this should be within a recurrent miscarriage clinic.

Detailed history:

- Gestation at miscarriage
- Past obstetric history
  - Gestation at delivery
  - IUFD
  - Painless dilatation of cervix/ruptured membranes
- History of thromboembolism
- Ultrasound confirmation of pregnancy
- Presence/absence of fetal heart on ultrasound
- Histological confirmation of products of conception in prior miscarriages.

Investigations and treatment

- Antiphospholipid antibodies
  - To diagnose APS, the woman should have two positive tests, at least 12 weeks apart, for either lupus anticoagulant or anticardiolipin antibodies of immunoglobulin G and/or immunoglobulin M
  - Pregnant women with APS should be treated with low-dose aspirin plus heparin to prevent further miscarriage. This treatment is initiated, in joint discussion with the haematologists. This treatment combination significantly reduces the miscarriage rate by >50%
- Chromosomal analysis of products of conception of third and subsequent consecutive miscarriages
- Karyotyping both partners
  - The finding of an abnormal parental karyotype should prompt referral to a clinical geneticist. Genetic counselling offers the couple a prognosis for the risk of future pregnancies with an unbalanced chromosome complement and the opportunity for familial chromosome studies
  - Reproductive options in couples with chromosomal rearrangements include proceeding to a further natural pregnancy, with or without a prenatal diagnosis test, gamete donation, and adoption
  - Preimplantation genetic diagnosis should be considered as an option for translocation carriers
- TVUS
  - To detect uterine anatomical abnormalities. Further investigations with 3-D scan, hysteroscopy, or laparoscopy may be required
  - However, there is insufficient evidence to assess the effect of uterine septum resection in women with recurrent miscarriage and uterine septum to prevent further miscarriage
- Investigations for PCOS

- Free testosterone, serum FSH and LH levels
  - However, there is insufficient evidence to advocate the use of progesterone or metformin in women with recurrent miscarriage
- Thrombophilia screen
  - Factor V Leiden, factor II (prothrombin) gene mutation, and protein S deficiency
  - There is insufficient evidence to evaluate the effect of heparin in pregnancy to prevent a miscarriage in women with recurrent first-trimester miscarriage associated with inherited thrombophilia
  - Heparin therapy during pregnancy may improve the live birth rate of women with second-trimester miscarriage associated with inherited thrombophilias
- Serial cervical sonographic surveillance or cervical cerclage may be offered to women with a history of second-trimester miscarriage where cervical weakness is suspected
- A significant proportion of cases of recurrent miscarriage remains unexplained despite detailed investigation. These women can be reassured that the prognosis for a successful future pregnancy with supportive care alone is in the region of 75%. However, prognosis does worsen with increasing age and number of previous miscarriages.

Further reading

Royal College of Obstetricians and Gynaecologists (2011). *The investigation and treatment of couples with recurrent first-trimester and second-trimester miscarriage*. Green-top guideline No. 17. Available at: <http://www.rcog.org.uk/files/rcog-corp/GTG17recurrentmiscarriage.pdf>.

Care pathway for recurrent miscarriage

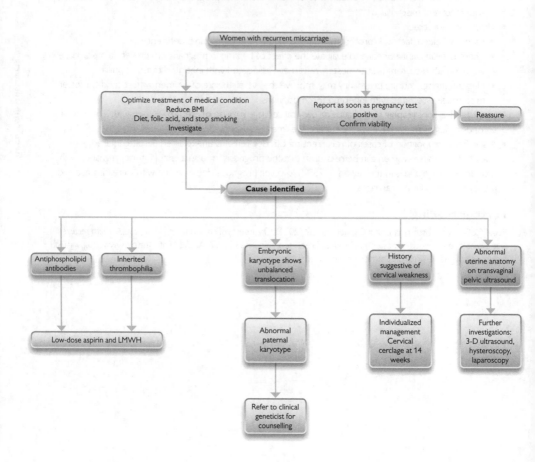

Trophoblastic disease

Key learning points

Gestational trophoblastic diseases (GTDs) include molar pregnancies and those with invasive potential, termed gestational trophoblastic neoplasia (GTN). The terms GTN and GTD are not interchangeable

All cases of GTD in the UK should be managed through the three dedicated centres

Even in advanced stages, GTN is usually curable due to the high sensitivity to chemotherapeutic agents

Surgical evacuation of the uterus, with avoidance of cervical preparation and oxytocic drugs, is the treatment of choice for suspected molar pregnancies.

Introduction

GTDs include a spectrum of interrelated tumours, including complete and partial hydatidiform mole. In addition, invasive mole, choriocarcinoma, and placental site trophoblastic tumour (PSTT) are also GTD but are termed GTN. Unusually, GTN can be cured, even in the presence of widespread metastases.

Molar pregnancy consists of two distinct entities, partial and complete moles, which can be distinguished by means of gross morphologic and histological examinations and according to chromosomal patterns.

In the UK, following a molar pregnancy, all monitoring and subsequent management is coordinated through three national referral centres.

Clinical significance

Hydatidiform moles are abnormal conceptions, occurring in 1:500–1000 pregnancies.

Risk factors

- Maternal age
- Previous history of molar pregnancy
- Geographical factors
- Ethnicity
- Paternal age.

Pathophysiology

Chromosomally deficient oocytes are fertilized by paternal sperm, either monospermic with duplication or dispermic. The resultant androgenetic conceptus will then have the 46 XX, 46 XY complement and will form the complete moles. The partial mole, however, retains the maternal component and is usually triploid, either from dispermic fertilization or from fertilization with an unreduced diploid sperm.

Clinical features

- Vaginal bleeding (commonest symptom)
- Excessive uterine enlargement
- Theca lutein cysts
- Hyperemesis gravidarum
- Pre-eclampsia
- Hyperthyroidism
- Rarely, neurological and respiratory symptoms.

Management

Ultrasound diagnosis of complete mole is characteristically described as having a snowstorm appearance, although many will be diagnosed as an incomplete/anembryonic pregnancy.

Partial mole may show a coexistent live fetus, with only scattered cystic spaces in the placenta. Characteristically, the diagnosis of partial mole is made after histological review of curettage specimens from presumed incomplete or missed abortions.

Quantitative serum β-hCG is elevated, usually >100 000 IU/L in the complete mole.

An FBC and liver and renal function tests should be obtained. Chest radiography, CT scan, or an MRI may be required to exclude metastatic spread.

Suction curettage is the preferred method for evacuation. Following primary treatment, patients are followed up with β-hCG assays to exclude residual disease.

Where suction curettage is performed for a suspected molar pregnancy, it is advised to avoid prostaglandin cervical preparation, oxytocic drugs, sharp curettage, or medical evacuation due to concerns that this may lead to dissemination of disease.

Gestational trophoblastic neoplasia

GTNs are malignant lesions that arise from abnormal proliferation of placental trophoblast and include:

- Invasive mole
- Choriocarcinoma
- PSTT
- Epithelioid trophoblastic tumour (ETT).

The main indicators are persistent vaginal bleeding and sustained elevation of β-hCG, following evacuation of a molar pregnancy.

The standardized International Federation of Gynecologists and Obstetricians (FIGO) hCG criteria for the diagnosis of post-molar GTD is well documented and include among others:

- Persistence of detectable hCG for >6 months after molar evacuation.

Using the FIGO scoring system (see Tables 1 and 2), GTN is divided into low-risk disease (scores <6) or high-risk disease (scores ≥7). High-risk GTN generally requires combination chemotherapy to achieve remission.

In low-risk disease, single-agent chemotherapy, using methotrexate, has been shown to achieve complete remission in >80% of cases. Alternatively, actinomycin D regimen has been shown to be as effective and can be used in patients with hepatic dysfunction or those with known adverse reactions to methotrexate.

Patients with high-risk disease are treated with combination chemotherapy. The EMACO regimen is preferred, as it has the best toxicity profile, with almost 100% complete remission rates.

Radiation and surgical adjuncts may be needed to treat stage IV high-risk disease.

Follow-up

The aims of follow-up are to confirm successful treatment and to identify women with persistent or malignant GTD who may require adjuvant chemotherapy or surgery at an early stage. Currently, 6 months' follow-up with hCG assays is recommended. This is coordinated from the referral centre.

Patients are advised to use effective contraception during follow-up. Hormonal contraception is not advised until hCG has normalized.

Table 1 FIGO anatomic staging for GTN

Stage I: disease confined to the uterus
Stage II: extends outside of the uterus but is limited to the genital structures (adnexa, vagina, broad ligament)
Stage III: extends to the lungs, with or without known genital tract involvement
Stage IV: all other metastatic sites

Reprinted from International Journal of Gynaecology and Obstetrics, 105, 1, FIGO Committee on Gynecologic Oncology, 'Current FIDO staging for cancer of the vagina, fallopian tube, ovary, and gestational trophoblastic neoplasia', pp. 3–4, copyright 2009, with permission from Elsevier and the International Federation of Gynaecology and Obstetrics.

Table 2 FIGO prognostic scoring system

Scores	0	1	2	4
Age (years)	≤39	≥40	–	–
Antecedent pregnancy	Mole	Abortion	Term	–
Interval from index pregnancy (months)	<4	4–6	7–12	>12
Pretreatment serum hCG (IU/L)	<1000	<10 000	<100 000	>100 000
Largest tumour size (including uterus)	–	3–4 cm	>5 cm	–
Site of metastases	Lung	Spleen/kidney	GI	Liver/brain
Number of metastases	–	1–4	5–8	>8
Previous failed chemotherapy	–	–	Single drug	2 or more

Reprinted from International Journal of Gynaecology and Obstetrics, 105, 1, FIGO Committee on Gynecologic Oncology, 'Current FIDO staging for cancer of the vagina, fallopian tube, ovary, and gestational trophoblastic neoplasia', pp. 3–4, copyright 2009, with permission from Elsevier and the International Federation of Gynaecology and Obstetrics.

Prognosis

Risk of recurrent molar pregnancy is 1:100. Fertility and pregnancy outcomes in women treated appear to be similar between those receiving single-agent and combination chemotherapy. The pregnancy outcomes also appeared similar to the normal population.

Further reading

Berkowitz RS and Goldstein DP (1997). Presentation and management of molar pregnancy. In BW Hancock, ES Newlands, RS Berkowitz, eds. Gestational trophoblastic disease, pp. 127–42. Chapman & Hall, London.

Berkowitz RS and Goldstein DP (2009). Molar pregnancy. New England Journal of Medicine, 360, 1639–45.

Bower M, Newlands ES, Holden L, et al. (1997). EMA/CO for high-risk gestational trophoblastic tumors: results from a cohort of 272 patients. Journal of Clinical Oncology, 15, 2636–43.

Cavaliere A, Ermito S, Dinatale A, Pedata R (2009). Management of molar pregnancy. Journal of Prenatal Medicine, 3, 15–17.

Kim S (1997). Epidemiology. In BW Hancock, ES Newlands, RS Berkowitz, eds. Gestational trophoblastic disease, pp. 27–42. Chapman & Hall, London.

Kohorn EI (2001). The new FIGO 2000 staging and risk factor scoring system for gestational trophoblastic disease: description and clinical assessment. International Journal of Gynecological Cancer, 11, 73–7.

May T, Goldstein DP, Berkowitz RS (2011). Current chemotherapeutic management of patients with gestational trophoblastic neoplasia. Chemotherapy Research and Practice, 2011, 806256.

Sebire NJ, Foskett M, Fisher RA, Rees H, Seckl M, Newlands E (2002). Risk of partial and complete hydatidiform molar pregnancy in relation to maternal age. British Journal of Obstetrics & Gynaecology, 109, 99–102.

Stone M and Bagshawe KD (1979). An analysis of the influences of maternal age, gestational age, contraceptive method, and the mode of primary treatment of patients with hydatidiform moles on the incidence of subsequent chemotherapy. British Journal of Obstetrics & Gynaecology, 86, 782–92.

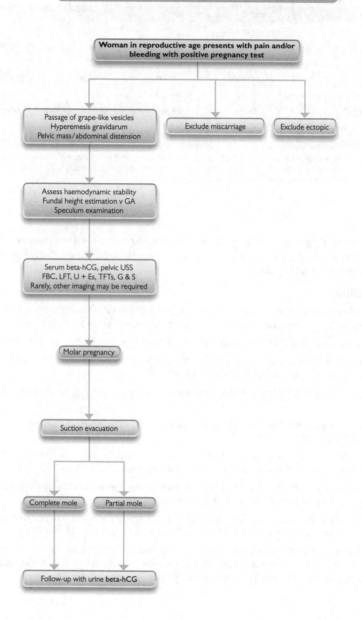

Care pathway for hydatidiform mole

Woman in reproductive age presents with pain and/or bleeding with positive pregnancy test

Passage of grape-like vesicles
Hyperemesis gravidarum
Pelvic mass/abdominal distension

Exclude miscarriage

Exclude ectopic

Assess haemodynamic stability
Fundal height estimation v GA
Speculum examination

Serum beta-hCG, pelvic USS
FBC, LFT, U + Es, TFTs, G & S
Rarely, other imaging may be required

Molar pregnancy

Suction evacuation

Complete mole

Partial mole

Follow-up with urine beta-hCG

Care pathway for gestational trophoblastic neoplasia

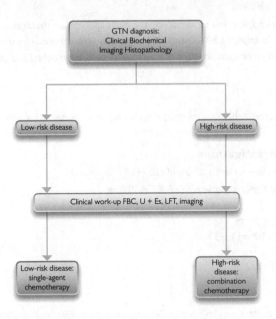

Management of the infertile couple

Key learning points

Investigation of the couple is key to identifying the most appropriate management strategy

Young couples should expect a 50% chance of conception with conservative management

Assisted conception techniques are part of a package of care, approached in a stepwise fashion.

Definition

Infertility is defined as the inability to conceive despite regular unprotected sexual intercourse (UPSI) for 2 years.

Aetiology and investigations

1. **Male factor:** responsible for around 30% of causes of infertility.

The criteria for normal semen parameters (WHO 2010) are:

Volume (mL): ≥1.5
Concentration (x 10^6 mL): ≥15
Total sperm number (x 10^6 mL): ≥39
Total motility (%): ≥40
Progressive motility (%): ≥32
Normal morphology (%): ≥4
WBC (x 10^6 mL): ≤1.

Abnormal semen parameters vary in severity. Genetic, endocrine, infectious, and lifestyle factors (such as smoking, excessive alcohol consumption, excessive stress, and obesity) varicoceles are identified causes of male subfertility. However, abnormal semen quality could be idiopathic in up to 50% of cases.

Causes for azoospermia (or absence of sperm in the ejaculate) are either obstructive, non-obstructive, or ejaculatory failure. The commonest causes for non-obstructive azoospermia are chromosomal abnormalities (including Y chromosome microdeletions), trauma, infections, and idiopathic. Congenital absence of the vas deferens is a common cause of obstructive azoospermia and is frequently associated with cystic fibrosis and renal malformations.

History, clinical examination, and semen analysis are basic investigations for male factor (see Algorithm).

2. **Ovulatory factor:** responsible for around 25% of causes of infertility.

A regular menstrual cycle is defined as a cycle occurring every 25–35 days. A mid-luteal progesterone level >28 nmol/L confirms normal ovulation.

The commonest causes of ovulatory dysfunction are PCOS, hypothalamic-pituitary dysfunction (such as excessive stress or exercise and pituitary tumours), and hypothroidism.

3. **Tubal factor:** responsible for around 15% of causes of infertility.

The commonest causes of tubal factor infertility are mainly caused by PID, previous pelvic surgery, and endo-metriosis. This can result in either blocked or patent pathological tubes. The commonly used tests for tubal patency are hysterosalpingogram, hysterocontrast sonography, and laparoscopy and dye test.

4. **Uterine factor:** responsible for around 5% of causes of infertility.

The commonest causes of uterine factor infertility are the presence of intrauterine adhesions, uterine septae, and submucous fibroids distorting the cavity. TVUS, hysterosalpingography, saline hysterosonography, and hysteroscopy are investigations to be considered.

5. **Unexplained infertility:** responsible for around 25% of causes of infertility.

It is a diagnosis made when no obvious cause is identified by routine investigations.

Ovarian reserve tests, such as anti-Müllerian hormone (AMH) and antral follicle count (AFC), may be helpful to predict ovarian response to ovarian stimulation prior to treatment.

A stepwise treatment approach is usually applied in these cases, but the treatment should be individualized, taking into account the result of ovarian reserve testing.

1. Expectant management: young couples with a short duration of unexplained infertility may expect a 50% chance of conception within 1 year with expectant management
2. Stimulated intrauterine insemination (IUI) and fallopian sperm perfusion
3. IVF
4. IVF with intracytoplasmic sperm injection (ICSI).

Acknowledgement

WHO criteria for normal semen parameters from Cooper TG, Noonan E, von Eckardstein S, et al. (2010) 'World Health Organization reference values for human semen characteristics', *Human Reproduction Update*, **16**, 3, pp. 231–245.

Further reading

National Institute for Health and Clinical Excellence (2013). *Fertility: assessment and treatment for people with fertility problem.* NICE clinical guideline 156. Available at: <http://guidance.nice.org.uk/CG156>.

Algorithm for male factor infertility

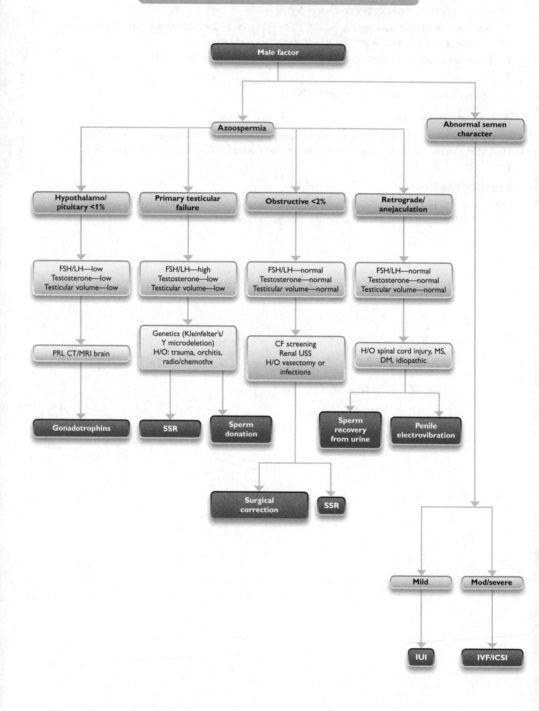

Algorithm for ovulatory disorders

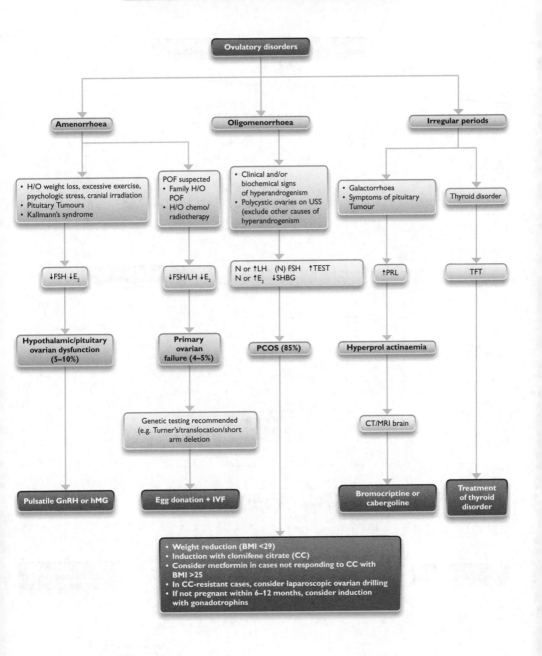

Algorithm for tubal factor

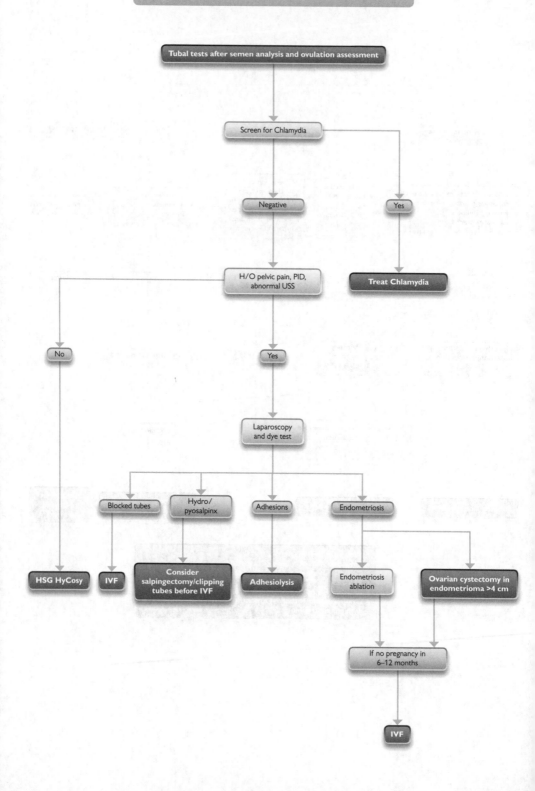

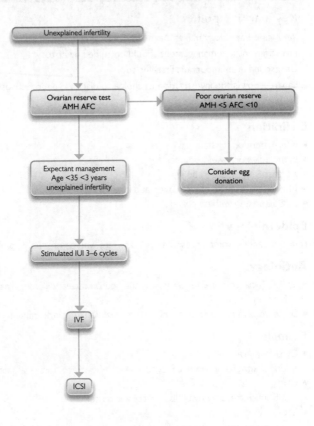

Chronic pelvic pain

Key learning points
Very varied aetiology makes diagnosis challenging
Investigations and management should be guided by history
Ultrasound is an important first-line tool
Laparoscopy is the investigation of choice to diagnose endometriosis.

Definition
- Intermittent or constant pain
- In the pelvis or lower abdomen
- At least 6 months' duration
- Not exclusively with menstruation and intercourse
- Not associated with pregnancy.

Epidemiology
Four per cent of women present to primary care with chronic pelvic pain.

Aetiology
- Various gynaecological, GI, urological, and neuromuscular disorders may cause or contribute to chronic pelvic pain
- Sometimes, multiple contributing factors may exist in a single patient.

Examples
- Gynaecological
  - Endometriosis, adhesions, PID, adnexal cysts, gynaecological malignancies, pelvic congestion syndrome
- GI
  - IBS, inflammatory bowel disease, colonic cancer
- Urological
  - Interstitial cystitis, chronic UTI, urolithiasis, bladder malignancy
- Musculoskeletal
  - Fibromyalgia, myofascial pain, degenerative disc disease
- Neurological
  - Trapped nerve, herpes zoster
- Psychiatric
  - Sleep disturbances, somatization, depression.

Presentation
Varied due to complex aetiology and the presence of associated disorders.

Management
History
- Important to explore patient's ideas, concerns, and expectations
- Multidisciplinary approach
- Thorough history is essential to direct further evaluation
- Detailed history of pain and systems essential.

Pain-specific history

- Location and distribution of pain
  - Use a pain diagram
  - Radiation important for neuropathic pain
- Nature of pain
  - Dull, colicky, burning, stabbing, shooting, throbbing
  - Colicky pain may indicated GI problems
  - Neurological pain may be burning
- Aggravating factors
  - Movement—musculoskeletal
  - Premenstrual—endometriosis
  - Specific diet—IBS
- Alleviating factors
  - Rest—musculoskeletal
- Associated factors
  - Depression, sleep deprivation
- Gynaecological and obstetric history
  - Menstrual history, abnormal vaginal bleeding, sexual abuse, multiple partners
- GI history
  - Change in bowel habit
- Urological history
  - Burning during micturition
- Past history
  - Previous surgery—adhesions.

Red flag symptoms

- Abnormal vaginal bleeding—irregular bleeding, intermenstrual bleeding, post-coital bleeding
- Rectal bleeding
- Change in bowel symptoms over 50 years
- Pelvic mass
- Unexplained weight loss
- Suicidal tendencies.

If history is suggestive of pain due to non-gynaecological component, referral to the relevant health care professional, such as gastroenterologist, GUM specialist, urologist, physiotherapist, psychologist, or psychosexual counsellor, should be considered.

Examination

- Guided by history
- Gynaecological examination
  - Abdominal examination—scars, masses, areas of tenderness
  - Speculum examination—discharge, appearance of cervix
  - Vaginal examination—size and shape of uterus; mobility; fornicial fullness, tenderness.

Investigations

TVUS

- Can diagnose adnexal pathologies, including endometriomas, other ovarian cysts, hydrosalpinges
- Adenomyosis
- Cannot diagnose peritoneal endometriotic deposits.

MRI pelvis

- Can diagnose adenomyosis
- Lacks sensitivity for endometriotic nodules but useful in the assessment of palpable nodules in the pelvis or when symptoms are suggestive of rectovaginal endometriosis
- MRI may also detect rare pathologies.

Laparoscopy

- Both a diagnostic as well as therapeutic intervention
- Only diagnostic test that can diagnose peritoneal endometriosis and adhesions
- Diagnostic laparoscopy has a role in developing a woman's beliefs about her pain.

Treatment

Cyclical pain

Women with cyclical pain benefit from the use of oral contraceptive pills, GnRh analogues, or IUS. A laparoscopy may be considered if a trial of 3–6 months does not help.

History or diagnostic laparoscopy suggestive of endometriosis

Therapeutic/operative laparoscopy by appropriately trained surgeon may be required.

Women with subfertility may need to be referred to fertility specialists.

History of prior surgeries, history of PID, adhesions on diagnostic laparoscopy

Operative laparoscopy for adhesiolysis may be required.

Symptoms suggestive of IBS

Consider treatment with antispasmodics, fibre diet, diet exclusion.

Further reading

Royal College of Obstetricians and Gynaecologists (2005). *The initial management of chronic pelvic pain*. Guideline No. 41. Available at: <http://www.rcog.org.uk/files/rcog-corp/uploaded-files/GT41InitialManagementChronicPelvic Pain2005.pdf>.

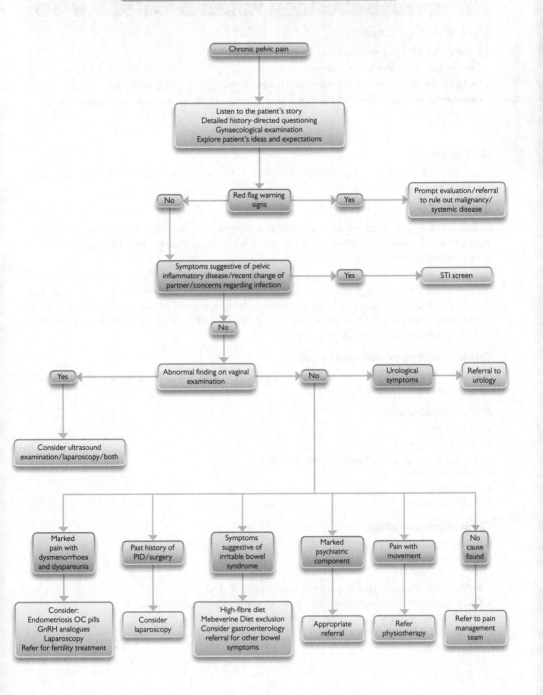

Care pathway for chronic pelvic pain

Chronic pelvic pain

Listen to the patient's story
Detailed history-directed questioning
Gynaecological examination
Explore patient's ideas and expectations

Red flag warning signs — No

Red flag warning signs — Yes → Prompt evaluation/referral to rule out malignancy/systemic disease

Symptoms suggestive of pelvic inflammatory disease/recent change of partner/concerns regarding infection — Yes → STI screen

No

Abnormal finding on vaginal examination — Yes

Abnormal finding on vaginal examination — No → Urological symptoms → Referral to urology

Consider ultrasound examination/laparoscopy/both

Marked pain with dysmenorrhoea and dyspareunia → Consider: Endometriosis OC pills GnRH analogues Laparoscopy Refer for fertility treatment

Past history of PID/surgery → Consider laparoscopy

Symptoms suggestive of irritable bowel syndrome → High-fibre diet Mebeverine Diet exclusion Consider gastroenterology referral for other bowel symptoms

Marked psychiatric component → Appropriate referral

Pain with movement → Refer physiotherapy

No cause found → Refer to pain management team

Endometriosis

Key learning points

Endometriosis is a chronic condition that tends to recur

Commonest sites are within the pelvis

Management within a multidisciplinary team is optimal management for severe cases

Laparoscopy with excision of affected areas is an effective diagnostic and treatment option, even in early disease.

Definition

Endometriosis is defined as a chronic condition in which there is growth of endometrial tissue in sites other than in the endometrial cavity.

Epidemiology

Overall, endometriosis affects between 6 and 20% of women, with a peak incidence at the age of 40. Further analysis of specific populations shows that the incidence is 20–30% of women with subfertility and 40–60% of women with dysmenorrhoea.

Endometriosis is a hormone-dependent process, and, whilst it can produce symptoms during the early reproductive years, it is more likely to present in women towards the end of their reproductive life as it spreads wider and develops complications, including endometriomata, invasive lesions, adhesions, and scarring. With the menopause, the natural history of endometriosis is a reduction of disease progression and invasion which is usually accompanied by a reduction in symptoms.

Common sites of endometriosis

Most cases of endometriosis involve lesions within the abdomen and pelvis. Other sites are much rarer, including lung, brain, skin, and scar tissue.

Abdominopelvic sites

- Peritoneum
- Pouch of Douglas
- In and around the ovaries, tubes, and ovarian fossae
- Bladder and urinary tract
- Rectovaginal space
- Within the bowel.

Clinical presentation

- Main symptoms
  - Dysmenorrhoea
  - Deep dyspareunia
  - Pelvic pain (chronic, with acute exacerbations upon ovulation)
- Other symptoms (often associated with longer-term or severe endometriosis)
  - Cyclical bowel-related pain, bloating, or bleeding
  - Cyclical bladder pain or haematuria
  - Subfertility
  - Chronic fatigue
  - Dyschezia.

Clinical findings

Examination, in most cases, of mild to moderate endometriosis may be normal. The main aim of examination is to establish the presence or absence of signs of more severe disease that may steer the immediate investigations and management. These signs include:

- Fixed point tenderness
  - Uterosacral ligaments
  - Overpalpable nodules
- A uterus with reduced mobility or fixed in its location
- Visible 'blue' nodules on the cervix or in the fornices
- Puckering at the vaginal vault
- Palpable nodules
  - In the rectovaginal septum
  - At the vaginal vault
- Pelvic mass.

Prior to examination of the patient suspected to have endometriosis, she should be warned that both the speculum and bimanual examination may be more uncomfortable than examination is normally and that, if an abnormality is found, she may require digital rectal examination. The clinician should take care to ensure the correct balance between obtaining enough information and causing pain.

Diagnosis

The optimal way to diagnose endometriosis is via laparoscopy, with histological confirmation, though patients should be informed that, if the disease is microscopic or very severe, a full assessment may be difficult.

Prior to laparoscopy, an ultrasound should be performed to exclude coexistent pathology such as endometriomata.

In cases where endometriomata, bowel, or bladder lesions are suspected or where surgery is planned, there is often value in performing an MRI which is often able to identify the following:

- Confirmation of cyst contents
- Demonstration of anatomical distortion that may signify adhesions
- Bladder or bowel invasion
- Ureteric blockade
- Rectovaginal fibrosis.

Serum CA-125 is usually raised in the presence of endometriosis but is not a diagnostic tool.

Specialist endometriosis assessment and management

If, on diagnostic laparoscopy, severe endometriosis is discovered, serious consideration should be given to the management of the patient at a centre with an established multidisciplinary team. This ensures enhanced patient safety and appropriateness of management. Appropriate disciplines required are:

- Radiology
- Colorectal surgery
- Urology
- Pain management
- Anaesthetics.

Management

- At all disease stages, appropriate analgesia should be used—with onward pain management referral, as needed
- If a diagnosis is suspected and the patient is happy, empirical treatment with simple hormonal therapy is appropriate
- Most other treatments should follow a laparoscopic diagnosis

- Hormonal therapy
  - Combined pill—effective when given normally or in a 'back-to-back' pattern
  - Progestogens
    - The 'mini pill', including newer progestogen contraceptives
    - Depot medroxyprogesterone acetate
    - Contraceptive implant
    - LNG-IUS
    - Danazol
  - GnRH agonists
    - Normally administered with tibolone as 'add back' to prevent hypoestrogenic adverse effects
    - Given following diagnosis in moderate to severe symptomatic cases
    - Not usually a long-term treatment; 6 months' therapy has been shown to improve pain and improve pregnancy rates
    - Useful to help plan suitability of proposed radical treatment
- Surgical
  - Should include excision, rather than 'point' diathermy of endometriotic lesions. Excision provides tissue for diagnosis, avoids diathermy necrosis of underlying organs, and is more effective
  - Most surgery should be completed laparoscopically, with total laparoscopic hysterectomy as the route of choice for women in whom hysterectomy is suitable
  - Fertility-preserving therapy
    - Drainage of endometriomata must include removal of the capsule
    - Division of adhesions
    - Excision of symptomatic plaques/lesions
  - Radical surgery
    - Oophorectomy
      - Unilateral to prevent recurrence in ovary with previous endometrioma
      - Bilateral to definitively treat the disease. Hysterectomy not essential
    - Excision of bladder/ureteric lesions must be performed with urology and fluoroscopy
    - Rectovaginal and other colorectal disease should be performed with colorectal surgeon. Laparoscopic route preferable, and patients should be preoperatively prepared for removal of sections of bowel and/or stoma
- Follow-up
  - Endometriosis is a chronic disease that will require follow-up, usually until the point of radical surgery or natural menopause
  - Patients who manage on simple therapies may be discharged to primary care but with a clear route back to specialist care planned
  - Chronic pain management and fertility input may also be required
  - Recurrence is common—between 20 and 50% after 5 years.

Further reading

Farquhar C (2007). Endometriosis. *BMJ*, **334**, 249–53.

Royal College of Obstetricians and Gynaecologists (2006). *The investigation and management of endometriosis.* Green-top guideline No. 24. Available at: <http://www.rcog.org.uk/files/rcog-corp/GTG2410022011.pdf>.

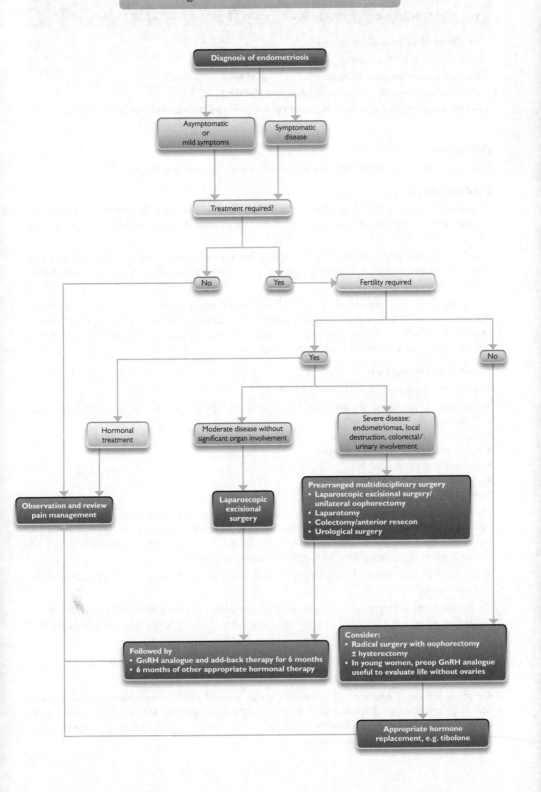

Algorithm for endometriosis

Diagnosis of endometriosis

Asymptomatic or mild symptoms

Symptomatic disease

Treatment required?

No

Yes

Fertility required

Yes

No

Hormonal treatment

Moderate disease without significant organ involvement

Severe disease: endometriomas, local destruction, colorectal/urinary involvement

Prearranged multidisciplinary surgery
- Laparoscopic excisional surgery/unilateral oophorectomy
- Laparotomy
- Colectomy/anterior resecon
- Urological surgery

Observation and review pain management

Laparoscopic excisional surgery

Followed by
- GnRH analogue and add-back therapy for 6 months
- 6 months of other appropriate hormonal therapy

Consider:
- Radical surgery with oophorectomy ± hysterectomy
- In young women, preop GnRH analogue useful to evaluate life without ovaries

Appropriate hormone replacement, e.g. tibolone

Fibroids

Key learning points

Fibroids are benign, hormone-dependent tumours

They are a common cause of pelvic mass and menorrhagia

Fibroids shrink after either natural, medical, or surgical menopause

Full counselling regarding treatment should take into account the patient's reproductive plans.

Definition

Fibroids (leiomyomata) are defined as benign tumours of myometrial smooth muscle.

Epidemiology

Fibroids are the commonest tumour of the female genital tract; their prevalence depends mainly upon the age at presentation and ethnicity, though other risk factors, such as nulliparity, obesity, alcohol intake, and a family history, should be considered.

It is difficult to obtain precise incidence figures; however, there is a cumulative incidence of approximately 30% in women between the ages of 25 and 45. Overall, the incidence of fibroids is 2–3-fold greater in black than in white women.

As fibroids are hormone-dependent tumours, they are more likely to present in women towards the end of their reproductive life as the fibroids grow. Black women have been shown to have clinically significant fibroids earlier in life than white women. Upon the onset of the menopause, the natural history of fibroids is to shrink, and this is usually accompanied by a reduction in symptoms.

Clinical presentation

Fibroids can present in any of the following scenarios:

- Asymptomatic pelvic mass, discovered incidentally at cervical screening or other opportunistic assessment
- Heavy menstrual bleeding (HMB)
- Pressure symptoms within the pelvis
- Subfertility and recurrent miscarriage
- Dysmenorrhoea
- Dyspareunia
- Acute pain.

The exact reasons behind the abnormal bleeding that often accompanies the presence of fibroids are not clearly understood. A submucous fibroid within the cavity may explain prolonged heavy periods, but it is harder to explain how the diffusely enlarged uterus can cause these symptoms. Explanations include an enlarged uterine cavity, dysregulated haemostasis, and abnormal vasculature.

Subfertility and miscarriage are thought to be due mainly to mechanical effects as a result of distortion of the uterus and cavity.

Rarely, fibroids can undergo an acute painful process such as torsion or degeneration. This is usually secondary to a permanent or temporary interruption in blood supply. A common cause of degeneration is pregnancy.

Diagnosis

When investigating fibroids thought to be responsible for HMB, it is important to ensure that other investigations for HMB are performed (see Chapter 53).

Abdominal and vaginal examination may establish the presence of a pelvic mass. Characteristically, this is a non-tender irregular mass that is normally mobile. Occasionally, during growth, the mass can become fixed in the sacral hollow, leading to pelvic pain and urinary symptoms. Occasionally, the uterus is so enlarged it can be difficult to distinguish from a pregnant uterus.

With ready access to modern imaging, it is important to confirm the diagnosis to ensure that other more serious forms of pelvic mass are not overlooked.

Ultrasound is readily available and a highly sensitive way of diagnosing the presence of fibroids. Due to the significant acoustic shadowing fibroids can cause, difficulties may be encountered in obtaining a complete assessment or a clear view of the endometrium. Thus, the use of MRI is increasingly used to obtain more thorough information to aid accurate diagnosis and plan treatment.

Hysteroscopy, preferably in the outpatient setting, is a useful tool for a thorough assessment of the impact of fibroids on the endometrial cavity. Modern hysteroscopic devices also provide an opportunity for treatment options in a 'one-stop' setting.

In most cases, histological analysis of an endometrial biopsy should be considered.

Treatment

- Watch and wait
  - As continued symptomatology from fibroids is dependent upon a premenopausal state, some patients (once investigated and a diagnosis is confirmed) are content to tolerate their symptoms and await natural menopause
- Medical treatments
  - In women with a diagnosis of HMB, menorrhagia thought to be caused by small fibroids may respond to non-hormonal symptomatic treatments such as NSAIDs (e.g. mefenamic acid) and antifibrinolytics (e.g. tranexamic acid)
  - Hormonal therapies, such as cyclical progestogens, COCP, and use of the LNG-IUS are useful early treatments. In some cases, it may be necessary to observe the uterine size to ensure that there is no growth in response to these exogenous hormones
  - GnRH agonists (GnRH-a) are the most effective way of shrinking fibroids and achieve up to 50% reduction in size. This shrinkage is most commonly used preoperatively to shrink fibroids and reduce operative complications. Due to the sudden menopause induced with these drugs, a form of hormone replacement (e.g. tibolone) may be given to ease symptoms and prevent bone loss without affecting fibroid shrinkage
  - A new oral treatment, ulipristal acetate, is a selective progesterone receptor modulator that appears to shrink fibroids. This recently released product is indicated for the preoperative treatment of fibroids only
- Surgical treatments
  - Resection of polyps within the cavity may improve menorrhagia symptoms and intermenstrual bleeding
  - Myomectomy (surgical excision of fibroids) may be performed as an open operation or laparoscopically. The greatest risk of this procedure is hysterectomy in approximately 5% of cases
- Interventional radiology
  - Uterine artery embolization under radiological control aims to permanently embolize fibroids or a portion of the uterus containing fibroids which results in permanent shrinkage due to fibroid necrosis. Data continue to be collected on this procedure, though it has achieved high popularity. Whilst fertility data after this procedure are not robust, there are reported cases of successful pregnancies. Further research is required
  - MRI-guided, focussed ultrasound fibroid ablation is a new procedure still within the research domain that involves a focussed ultrasound energy beam using MRI to plot where the fibroids are located. The beam heats the fibroids which results in local necrosis and subsequent shrinkage. Early reports are encouraging.

Conclusion

Fibroids, whilst benign tumours, can produce significant symptoms, with long-term irreversible consequences. Equally though, their presence in asymptomatic women should not be of immediate concern. There is now a wide range of treatment options to consider which require the patient's carer to be up to date with all possible management strategies to enable a fully informed choice of care pathway.

Further reading

National Institute for Health and Clinical Excellence (2007). *Heavy menstrual bleeding: investigation and treatment.* NICE clinical guideline 44. Available from <www.nice.org.uk/CG044>.

National Institute for Health and Clinical Excellence (2010). *Uterine artery embolisation for fibroids.* NICE interventional procedure guideline 367. Available at: <http://guidance.nice.org.uk/IPG367>.

Algorithm for fibroids

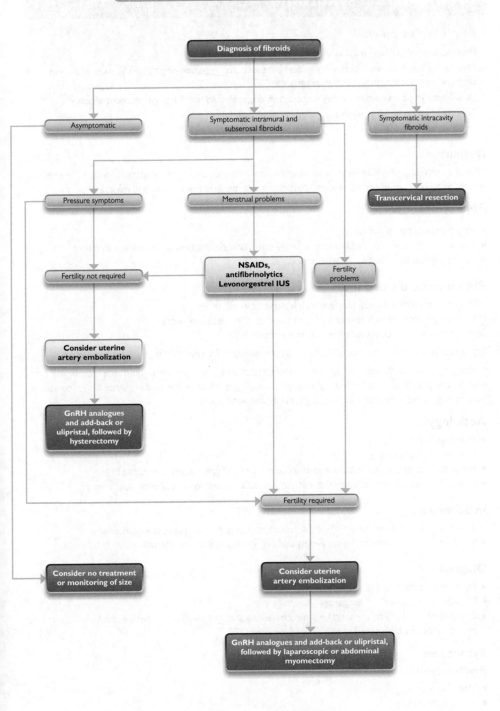

Premenstrual syndrome

Key learning points

Presentation of premenstrual syndrome (PMS) is very variable

One of the key features is that women feel best just after a period or at times in their life when they are not menstruating, such as pregnancy

Well-kept symptom diaries are key to accurate diagnosis and monitoring treatment efficacy

Treatment of underlying psychopathology is often helpful.

Definition

PMS is a distressing condition with physical, behavioural, and psychological symptoms, including depression, anxiety, irritability, loss of confidence, and physical symptoms, including bloating and mastalgia.

PMS symptoms

- Vary from woman to woman
- Occur prior to a period, usually improve at the onset of menstruation, and disappear by its end
- Women feel at their best just after a period.

PMS may be divided into:

Mild: symptoms which do not interfere with lifestyle or work

Moderate: symptoms which interfere with, but do not stop, lifestyle or work

Severe: symptoms which prevent interaction and work.

Premenstrual dysphoric disorder (PDD) is an alternative term for severe PMS.

Underlying psychopathology is suggested when symptoms continue throughout the menstrual cycle, even in the presence of premenstrual exaggeration. Bipolar disorders may sometimes be recognized by post-menstrual rebound into a state of high activity and exhilaration.

Aetiology

- Aetiology unknown
- Linked with ovarian cycle
- Probable association with neurotransmitters (serotonin and gamma-amino butyric acid)
- Association with obesity, less exercise, salt, alcohol, caffeine, and lower academic achievement.

Incidence

- 95% of women of reproductive age experience symptoms attributable to the ovarian cycle
- 5–10% have severe, debilitating symptoms that prevent normal activity/lifestyle.

Diagnosis

- No hormone abnormality
- No appropriate specific investigations
- The diagnosis is made by prospective symptom diaries and by identifying a repetitive relationship with the menstrual cycle (daily record of severity of problems, DRPS).

Symptoms

Psychological

- Mood swings
- Irritability/aggression
- Depression/tears.

Behavioural

- Inability to cope
- Poor cognitive ability
- Clumsiness/accidents.

Physical

- Bloating
- Headaches/migraines
- Breast tenderness
- Fatigue
- Food cravings
- Exacerbations of diseases, e.g. asthma, herpetic infection.

Management

- The impact of symptoms on lifestyle is used to judge the severity of PMS
- Underlying psychiatric or psychological problems should be excluded
- There appears to be some relationship between PMS, post-natal depression, menopausal symptoms, and seasonal affective disorder (SAD).

General advice about exercise, diet, and stress is always advisable. Those patients with underlying psychopathology should be managed with the help of a psychiatrist.

Treatments

Accurate assessment of success is only possible through the sustained use of daily records of symptoms and their severity (see Algorithm).

Complementary therapies

These include lifestyle/alternative therapies/vitamins and supplements/herbal remedies.

A large number of complementary medicines have been used for the treatment of PMS, but there is limited clinical evidence. Considerably more research is required before recommendations can be made.

Psychological therapies

Cognitive behavioural therapy appears to be effective, its benefits sustained, and should be considered for all those with severe, life-influencing PMS.

Medical

Selective serotonin reuptake inhibitors (SSRIs) and serotonin noradrenaline reuptake inhibitors (SNRIs) have been shown to significantly reduce symptoms. The new SSRIs, such as citalopram, appear to be more effective. Luteal treatment may be of greater benefit than continual medication and is associated with less risk of problem at withdrawal.

Hormone treatment

Combined contraceptives

The newer types of contraceptive pills containing better tolerated progestogens, e.g. drospirenone, should be considered as a first-line treatment of PMS. Continuous therapy, without a week free of medication, appears to be advantageous.

High-dosage oestrogen therapy

Percutaneous oestradiol, as high-dose patches (100–200 micrograms), is effective for the management of both the physical and psychological symptoms of severe PMS. The addition of a progestogen for endometrial protection may cause side effects which are PMS-like in character. The use of micronized progesterone or an LNG-IUS may be better tolerated.

Bromocriptine, tamoxifen, and danazol

May be helpful for women with severe breast pain, but danazol in particular is associated with a high risk of side effects.

GnRH analogues

GnRH analogue treatment is the 'gold standard therapy' for severe PMS. Continuing symptoms, despite GnRH treatment, suggests underlying psychopathology.

Although licensed for only 6 months' use, because of the associated risk of osteopenia, add-back therapy with tibolone (or continuous oestrogen and progestogen) allows longer-duration therapy. Add-back therapy preserves bone and eases vasomotor flushes, which can otherwise be profound. Regular bone density studies are recommended if GnRH treatment is used beyond 6 months.

Progestogens and progesterone

Evidence gives no support to the use of progestogens for the treatment of PMS which may themselves cause PMS-like symptoms. Progesterone appears to cause fewer side effects and have possible advantages in terms of acting as a diuretic and anxiolytic. Larger studies are required.

Surgical

(Hysterectomy and) bilateral oophorectomy

Bilateral oophorectomy is a definitive and permanent method of ovarian cycle suppression.

Successful treatment of PMS, using a GnRH analogue, is a prerequisite before considering surgical oophorectomy.

Oophorectomy is infrequently required but sometimes preferred as a long-term strategy once childbearing is complete. For climacteric symptom relief and bone protection, HRT is recommended after oophorectomy. HRT should be recommended to continue to, at least, the age of 50 years.

Hysterectomy, at the same time as an oophorectomy, allows oestrogen-only replacement therapy (ERT) that, in the absence of a progestogen, is less likely to cause side effects and is possibly safer.

Further reading

Endicott J, Nee J, Harrison W (2006). Daily record of severity of problems (DRSP): reliability and validity. Archives of Women's Mental Health, 8, 41–9.

Royal College of Obstetricians and Gynaecologists (2007). Management of premenstrual syndrome. Green-top guideline No. 48. Available at: <http://www.rcog.org.uk/files/rcog-corp/uploaded-files/GT48ManagementPremensturalSyndrome.pdf>.

Care pathway for premenstrual syndrome

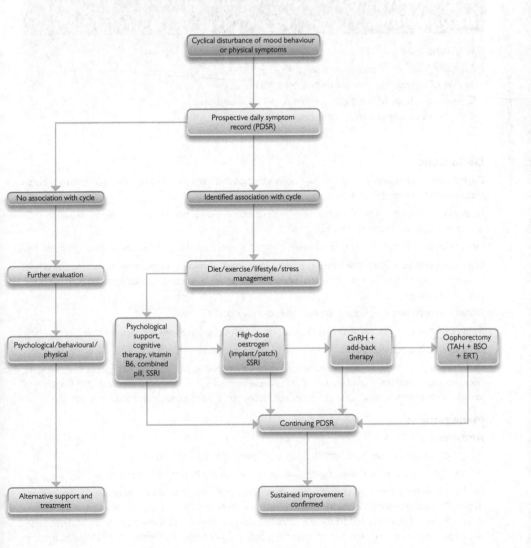

Urinary urgency, frequency, and urinary incontinence

Key learning points

Adequate history of high importance

Conservative treatment should be first line of management

Consider urodynamic investigation when surgery contemplated

Complex cases may require multidisciplinary input

Definitions

Daytime urinary frequency is the complaint of micturition that occurs more frequently during waking hours than previously deemed normal by the woman.

Nocturia is the complaint of interruption of sleep one or more times because of the need to micturate. Each void is preceded and followed by sleep.

Urinary urgency is the complaint of a sudden, compelling desire to pass urine, which is difficult to defer.

Overactive bladder (OAB) syndrome involves urinary urgency, usually accompanied by frequency and nocturia, with or without urinary urgency incontinence, in the absence of a urinary tract infection (UTI) or other obvious pathology.

Urinary incontinence (UI) is the complaint of involuntary loss of urine.

Stress UI is the complaint of involuntary loss of urine on effort or physical exertion, or on sneezing or coughing.

Urgency UI is the complaint of involuntary loss of urine, associated with urgency.

Other types of UI are postural incontinence, nocturnal enuresis (involuntary urinary loss of urine during sleep), mixed incontinence (involuntary loss of urine associated with urgency and also with effort or physical exertion or on sneezing or coughing), continuous incontinence, and insensible and coital incontinence.

Management

Assessment

A urine dipstick test is used to detect blood, glucose, protein, leucocytes, and nitrites.

A bladder diary for at least 3 days, covering variations in usual activities, should be completed.

For the few women with pure stress UI, multichannel cystometry is not routinely necessary before primary surgery. Multichannel filling and voiding cystometry, and ambulatory urodynamics or videourodynamics before surgery for UI are recommended if there is clinical suspicion of detrusor overactivity, or there has been previous surgery for stress UI or anterior compartment prolapse, or there are symptoms of voiding dysfunction.

Treatment

Lifestyle interventions

Women with UI or OAB should be advised to modify fluid intake and lose weight if their BMI is >30.

Pelvic floor muscle training (PFMT) for at least 3 months is the first-line treatment for stress or mixed UI.

Stress UI

If conservative treatments have failed, treatment options include retropubic or transobturator mid-urethral tape insertion, with macroporous (type 1) polypropylene mesh, open colposuspension, or autologous rectus fascial sling.

Intramural bulking agents can be used; however, repeat injections may be needed; the effect decreases over time, and the technique is less effective than retropubic suspension or sling.

An artificial urinary sphincter may be an option if previous surgery has failed.

Mixed UI

Treatment should be tailored, according to the dominant symptom.

OAB with or without urge UI

Caffeine reduction and bladder training, lasting at least 6 weeks, are first-line treatments for urgency or mixed UI. If symptoms persist, an antimuscarinic drug can be prescribed (oxybutynin, darifenacin, solifenacin, tolterodine, fesoterodine, trospium, mirabegron, or different oxybutynin formulations). Mirabegron is a selective beta3 adrenoceptor agonist and is an option for treating the symptoms of OAB for people in whom antimuscarinic drugs are contraindicated or clinically ineffective, or have unacceptable side effects. Desmopressin may be used to reduce troublesome nocturia. In post-menopausal women with vaginal atrophy, intravaginal oestrogens may be effective for OAB symptoms. If conservative treatments have failed, botulinum toxin A may be considered, but the high risk of post-operative voiding dysfunction and requirement for chronic catheterization or self-catheterization should be discussed.

Sacral nerve stimulation and posterior tibial nerve stimulation are alternative treatment options for selected women with refractory OAB.

In women with severe OAB and significant impairment of quality of life, augmentation cystoplasty or urinary diversion are surgical treatments with common and serious complications.

Further reading

Haylen BT, de Ridder D, Freeman RM, et al. (2010). An International Urogynecological Association (IUGA)/ International Continence Society (ICS) joint report on the terminology for female pelvic floor dysfunction. International Urogynecological Journal, **21**, 5–26.

Lucas MG, Bosch JLHR, Cruz F, et al.; European Association of Urology (2012). Guidelines on urinary incontinence. Available at: <http://www.uroweb.org/gls/pdf/18_Urinary_Incontinence_LR.pdf>.

National Institute for Health and Clinical Excellence (2013). Urinary incontinence. The management of urinary incontinence in women. Available at: <http://guidance.nice.org.uk/CG171>.

Algorithm for urinary urgency, frequency, and incontinence

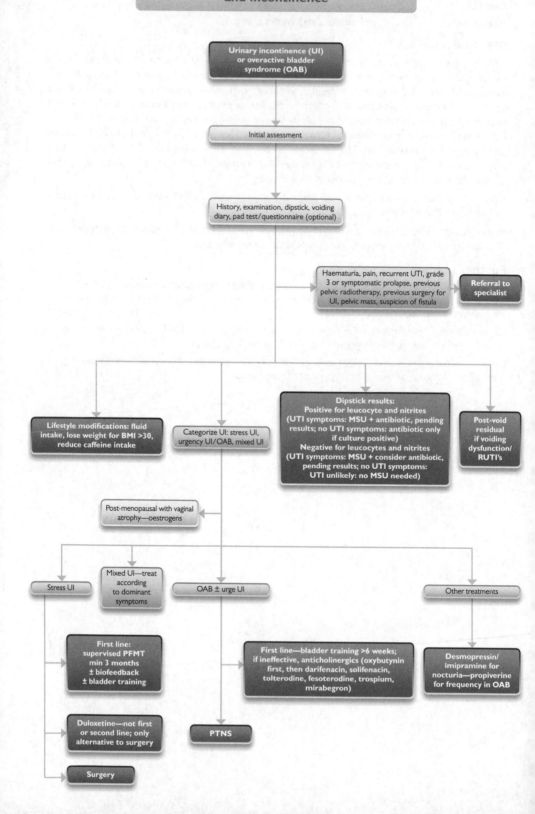

Urinary incontinence (UI) or overactive bladder syndrome (OAB)

Initial assessment

History, examination, dipstick, voiding diary, pad test/questionnaire (optional)

Haematuria, pain, recurrent UTI, grade 3 or symptomatic prolapse, previous pelvic radiotherapy, previous surgery for UI, pelvic mass, suspicion of fistula

Referral to specialist

Lifestyle modifications: fluid intake, lose weight for BMI >30, reduce caffeine intake

Categorize UI: stress UI, urgency UI/OAB, mixed UI

Dipstick results:
Positive for leucocyte and nitrites
(UTI symptoms: MSU + antibiotic, pending results; no UTI symptoms: antibiotic only if culture positive)
Negative for leucocytes and nitrites
(UTI symptoms: MSU + consider antibiotic, pending results; no UTI symptoms: UTI unlikely: no MSU needed)

Post-void residual if voiding dysfunction/ RUTI's

Post-menopausal with vaginal atrophy—oestrogens

Stress UI

Mixed UI—treat according to dominant symptoms

OAB ± urge UI

Other treatments

First line: supervised PFMT min 3 months ± biofeedback ± bladder training

First line—bladder training >6 weeks; if ineffective, anticholinergics (oxybutynin first, then darifenacin, solifenacin, tolterodine, fesoterodine, trospium, mirabegron)

Desmopressin/ imipramine for nocturia—propiverine for frequency in OAB

Duloxetine—not first or second line; only alternative to surgery

PTNS

Surgery

Algorithm for urinary urgency, frequency, and incontinence

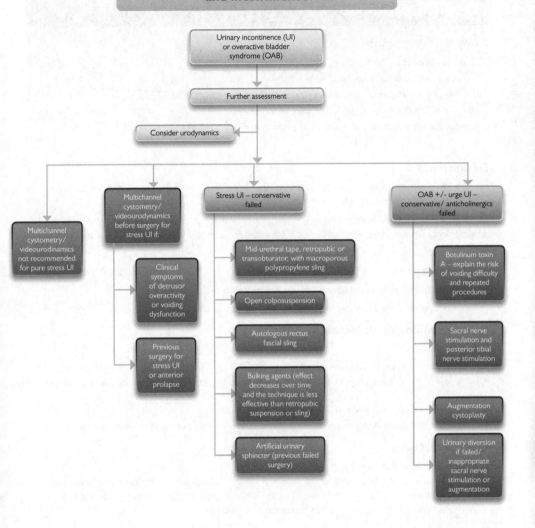

Urinary incontinence (UI) or overactive bladder syndrome (OAB)

Further assessment

Consider urodynamics

Multichannel cystometry/ videourodinamics not recommended for pure stress UI

Multichannel cystometry/ videourodynamics before surgery for stress UI if:

Clinical symptoms of detrusor overactivity or voiding dysfunction

Previous surgery for stress UI or anterior prolapse

Stress UI – conservative failed

Mid-urethral tape, retropubic or transobturator, with macroporous polypropylene sling

Open colposuspension

Autologous rectus fascial sling

Bulking agents (effect decreases over time and the technique is less effective than retropubic suspension or sling)

Artificial urinary sphincter (previous failed surgery)

OAB +/- urge UI – conservative/ anticholinergics failed

Botulinum toxin A – explain the risk of voiding difficulty and repeated procedures

Sacral nerve stimulation and posterior tibial nerve stimulation

Augmentation cystoplasty

Urinary diversion if failed/ inappropriate sacral nerve stimulation or augmentation

Genital prolapse

Key learning points

Common condition, with a significant impact on quality of life

Genetic predisposition associated with prolapse

Correlation of symptoms with anatomical changes during clinical assessment

Lifestyle modification is an important part of treatment

Careful patient selection and counselling prior to surgery to minimize recurrence.

Definition

Pelvic organ prolapse is defined as the descent of the pelvic organs into the vagina, often accompanied by urinary, bowel, sexual, or local pelvic symptoms.

Demographic changes with increasing longevity, rising patient expectations, increasing awareness, and the development of novel treatment techniques means that prevalence will continue to rise in the foreseeable future.

Epidemiology

The true incidence is unknown, but prevalence rates range from 25 to 65%.

Prolapse represents a significant cause of morbidity to individuals and a significant burden on health services.

Pathophysiology/risk factors

Risk factors include:

- Personal attributes such as age, menopausal state, and ethnicity (Caucasian race)
- Potentially modifiable aetiologic factors include parity, obesity, lifestyle factors such as smoking and heavy lifting
- Genetic factors, including Ehlers–Danlos syndrome
- Obstetric factors such as macrosomia, prolonged second stage of labour, and obstetric trauma.

Clinical features

- Prolapse can be asymptomatic
- Symptomatic women may present with a variety of symptoms (vaginal, urinary, bowel, back pain, and sexual symptoms). Vaginal symptoms, like sensation of, or seeing, a bulge, is believed to be the only specific symptom. Other symptoms can be unrelated to prolapse.

Examination

- Ideally carried out in the left lateral position with a Sims speculum
- Assess presence or absence of vulval atrophy
- The vaginal walls, including the vaginal apex, and the cervix should be systematically examined, while the patient is asked to strain, to assess the extent of descent
- If appropriate, also examine in standing position.

Various grading systems for quantifying the degree of prolapse are available, including the traditional severity grading—the POP-Q system, the Baden–Walker system, and a combination of POP-Q and Baden–Walker systems.

Management

Expectant management

- Evidence exists that prolapse may itself regress. Lifestyle intervention that acts by decreasing abdominal pressure, e.g. avoiding heavy lifting, weight reduction, and smoking cessation, helps symptom alleviation.

The mainstay of management involves conservative and surgical interventions.

The main goal of treatment should be the relief of patient symptoms and restoration of function, rather than the achievement of clinically defined anatomic landmarks.

The two major treatment options are conservative and surgical—they are not mutually exclusive.

Conservative treatment

Pessaries

Proven efficacy in the relief of prolapse symptoms. Common indications:

- Preference for non-surgical management
- Poor surgical risk
- As a temporary method, while planning definitive surgery, or until childbearing is completed.

Pelvic floor muscle training

- Effective in early stages of prolapse
- Symptomatic improvement is usually short-lived.

Surgical management

- There are established procedures for repair of prolapse of specific compartments
- The vaginal route remains the preferred option
- Abdominal, laparoscopic, and robotic routes can all be used
- Vaginal and laparoscopic routes of surgery have less morbidity than abdominal surgery
- Primary repairs are commonly performed using native tissues. Augmentation for reinforcement of repair is still evolving. There is still debate as to the utility of meshes and biological grafts for primary or secondary repairs, due to concerns about the complications of meshes, including pain, erosions, and mesh contracture
- Vault suspension with hysterectomy, using a variety of techniques, is recommended, as simple hysterectomy will not correct prolapse
- Consent for these procedures should highlight the risk of reoperation due to various factors. The risk of recurrence following surgical repairs can be as high as 30%.

Conclusion

Genital prolapse has a diverse presentation, with significant impact on patients' quality of life.
Tailored to individual diagnosis, management must be carefully targeted, with the ultimate aim being to alleviate symptoms and restore function with the minimal morbidity.

Further reading

Brubaker L, Glazener C, Jacquelin B, et al. (2009). Surgery for pelvic organ prolapse. In P Abrams, L Cardozo, S Khoury, A Wein, eds. Incontinence, pp. 1273–320. Health Publication Ltd, Plymouth.

Doshani A, Teo REC, Mayne CJ, Tincello DG (2007). Uterine prolapse. BMJ, **335**, 819–23.

Machin SM and Mukhopadhyay S (2011). Pelvic organ prolapse: review of the aetiology, presentation, diagnosis and management. Menopause International, **17**, 132–6.

Swift S, Woodman P, O'Boyle A, et al. (2005). Pelvic organ support study (POSST): the distribution, clinical definition and epidemiologic condition of pelvic organ support defects. American Journal of Obstetrics & Gynecology, **192**, 795–806.

Algorithm for genital prolapse

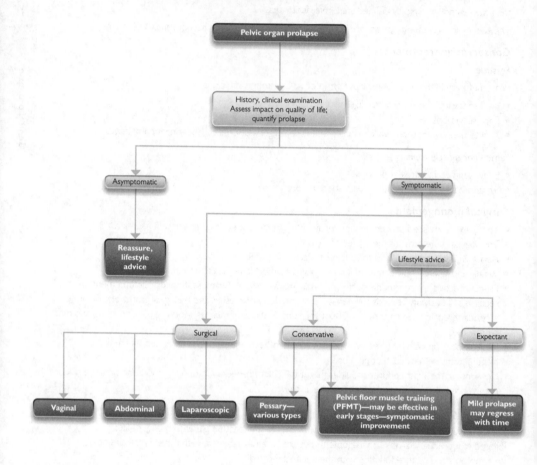

Post-menopausal bleeding

Key learning points

Post-menopausal bleeding (PMB) is a common symptom of gynaecological malignancy

One-stop use of transvaginal scanning (TVS), endometrial biopsy, and, where appropriate, hysteroscopy is considered optimal assessment.

Definition

An episode of bleeding 12 months or more after the last menstrual period. In addition, unscheduled bleeding, whilst taking HRT, should be investigated as for PMB.

Background

Approximately 10% of patients presenting with PMB will have a gynaecological malignancy. Since 80–90% of patients with endometrial cancer experience abnormal bleeding, the vast majority of patients with malignancy presenting as PMB will be endometrial in origin. There will, however, be occasional cases of cervical, vaginal, vulval, and ovarian cancer which are referred with PMB.

History and examination

A comprehensive history should be taken, in particular, risk factors for endometrial hyperplasia/cancer:

- Obesity
- Hypertension
- Diabetes
- Tamoxifen
- Nulliparity
- Late menopause.

Examination should include assessment of the entire lower genital tract, as many patients with PMB will have a non-endometrial cause for bleeding, e.g. atrophic vaginitis.

Causes of post-menopausal bleeding

- Atrophic vaginitis
- Endometrial cancer/hyperplasia
- Cervical cancer
- Vulval cancer
- Vaginal cancer (rare)
- Ovarian/Fallopian tube cancer (rare presenting symptom)
- Cervical polyps.

Investigation

Ultrasound

TVS is most accurate; transabdominal assessment only if TVS is not possible.

TVS must be performed before attempting endometrial sampling, as this may affect the appearance of the endometrium.

Risk of endometrial cancer is related to the endometrial thickness (ET), with the incidence of endometrial cancer in women with ET <4 mm being rare (0.6%).

The sensitivity of TVS for the detection of polyps is poor, with an incidence of 34, 64, and 61% for ET of 5–8, 9–12, and >12 mm, respectively. In patients in whom a polyp is suspected on TVS, the incidence is 55%. Hysteroscopy is indicated if ET is >10 mm.

Measurement of ET may not be possible due to fibroids or endometrial pathology causing the endometrium to be isoechoic with the myometrium.

The pelvic ultrasound report should note:

- ET (measuring the anteroposterior two-layer thickness in the sagittal plane near the fundus)
- Suspected polyps
- Uterine size
- Ovarian morphology
- Presence of fibroids
- Presence of ascites.

Endometrial biopsy

Indications

ET ≥4 mm
ET not visualized, e.g. fibroids
Recurrent PMB, regardless of ET

An endometrial sampling device (e.g. Pipelle TM) should be used; this provides a sensitivity of 99% and 88%, respectively, for the detection of endometrial cancer and atypical endometrial hyperplasia in post-menopausal women.

Using an ET of ≥4 mm a sensitivity of 95% and specificity of 55% are obtained. Therefore, patients presenting with PMB for the first time with an ET <4 mm do not require an endometrial biopsy.

In view of the 5% false negative rate with an ET <4 mm, an endometrial biopsy should be obtained in all patients presenting with recurrent PMB, regardless of the ET.

Hysteroscopy

Indications

Unable to pass endometrial sampler
ET >10 mm or suspected polyp on USS
Inadequate visualization of endometrium
Inadequate Pipelle biopsy
Recurrent PMB.

Note that hysteroscopy should not be performed until the results of the Pipelle biopsy are known, since the result may obviate the need for further investigation, e.g. endometrial cancer or atypical endometrial hyperplasia.

Outpatient hysteroscopy is preferred.

Further reading

Baiocchi G, Manci N, Pazzaglia M, et al. (2009). Malignancy in endometrial polyps: a 12-year experience. American Journal of Obstetrics & Gynecology, 201, 462 e1–4.

Dijkhuizen FP, Mol BW, Brolmann HA, Heintz AP (2000). The accuracy of endometrial sampling in the diagnosis of patients with endometrial carcinoma and hyperplasia: a meta-analysis. Cancer, 89, 1765–72.

Dubinsky TJ (2004). Value of sonography in the diagnosis of abnormal vaginal bleeding. Journal of Clinical Ultrasound, 32, 348–53.

Timmermans A, Gerritse MB, Opmeer BC, Jansen FW, Mol BW, Veersema S (2008). Diagnostic accuracy of endometrial thickness to exclude polyps in women with postmenopausal bleeding. Journal of Clinical Ultrasound, 36, 286–90.

Algorithm for post-menopausal bleeding

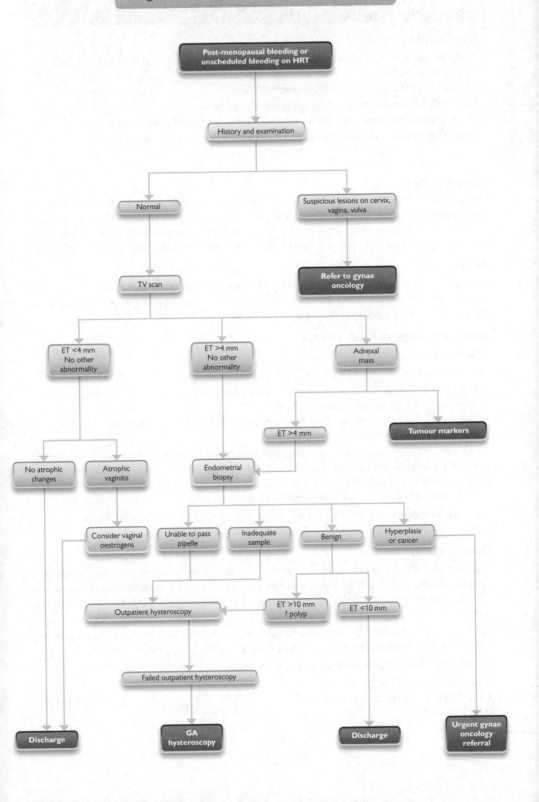

Gynaecological cancers

Key learning points

Whilst incidence for cervical and ovarian cancers have decreased, that of endometrial and vulval cancers has increased

Obesity is a significant risk factor for endometrial cancer

Ovarian cancer tends to present late, with poor survival rates

There is no effective screening modality for endometrial, ovarian, or vulval cancers

Surgery remains the main treatment option for gynaecological malignancies.

Epidemiology

Uterine cancer is the fourth most common cancer diagnosed in women in the UK. In 2008, 7703 new cases were diagnosed, accounting for 5% of all female malignancies. During the same period, 6537 new cases of ovarian cancer were diagnosed, comprising 4.2% of all female cancers (excluding non-melanoma skin cancer). The respective figures for cervical, vulval, and vaginal malignancies were 2938 (1.9%), 1157 (0.8%), and 258 (0.2%).

Trends

In the last decade, an increase has been observed in the age-standardized incidence rate for endometrial and vulval cancer (increase of 27% and 8%, respectively). However, the age-standardized rate for ovarian and cervical cancer has decreased in the last decade (12% for each type of cancer).

Histopathology and risk factors

Uterine cancer

Two types of uterine cancer are recognized:

- Type I tumours comprise 80% of the cases and have endometrioid histology. The most common histological type is endometrioid adenocarcinoma
- Type II tumours account for only 20% and have non-endometrioid histology, most commonly, clear cell or papillary serous carcinoma.

Type I uterine tumours are associated with unopposed oestrogen stimulation of the endometrium. Risk factors for the development of type I endometrial carcinoma include increasing age, obesity, presence of diabetes or hypertension, use of tamoxifen, or a history of breast cancer and genetic mutations (Lynch syndrome). Type I tumours are often preceded by endometrial hyperplasia.

In contrast, women with type II tumours have no recognized risk factors or precursor lesions. These tumours show an association with obesity, but this is less pronounced that for type I malignancies.

Ovarian cancer

Approximately 90% of ovarian tumours originate from the surface epithelium, and the most common subtypes include serous, mucinous, and endometrioid histology. Ovarian sex cord stromal tumours develop from the cells surrounding the oocyte and include granulosa cell, fibroma, thecoma, Sertoli cell, and Sertoli-Leydig tumours.

Germ cell tumours develop from the primordial germ cells of the ovary, and histological types include teratoma, dysgerminoma, choriocarcinoma, embryonal carcinoma, and yolk sac tumours.

Risk factors for developing epithelial ovarian carcinoma include:

- Nulliparity
- Family history of breast or ovarian cancer
- Early menarche

- Late menopause
- White race
- Increasing age
- Personal history of breast cancer
- Ethnic background (Ashkenazi Jewish families)
- *BRCA* gene mutations.

Cervical cancer

In the UK, squamous cell carcinomas account for approximately two-thirds of cervical cancer cases, adenocarcinoma for 15%, and a further 15% are poorly specified carcinomas.

HPV is detected in 99.7% of cases of cervical cancer and is the most important factor for development of cervical cancer.

Other risk factors include:

- Early onset of sexual activity
- Multiple sexual partners
- Smoking
- Immunosuppression
- Prolonged use of oral contraceptives
- High parity
- Low socio-economic status.

Vulval cancer

Squamous cell carcinoma is the most common histological type of vulval malignancy. Other histopathological types of vulval malignancies include melanoma (second most common type), basal cell carcinoma, sarcoma, extramammary Paget's disease, and Bartholin's gland adenocarcinoma.

Risk factors for vulval cancer include:

- HPV infection
- Chronic inflammatory or autoimmune conditions of the vulva (e.g. lichen sclerosus)
- Smoking
- Vulval intraepithelial neoplasia
- Immunosuppression.

Vaginal cancer

Up to 80% of vaginal tumours are squamous cell carcinomas, 14% adenocarcinomas, and the remaining 6–7% are melanomas and sarcomas.

Vaginal cancer, similarly to cervical cancer, is associated with:

- HPV infection
- Smoking
- Multiple sexual partners.

Clear cell carcinoma is more commonly diagnosed in women exposed to diethylstilboestrol (DES) *in utero*.

Clinical presentation

The majority of cases of endometrial cancer are diagnosed in post-menopausal women. Post-menopausal vaginal bleeding is the most common presenting symptom. Other symptoms include irregular perimenopausal bleeding or vaginal discharge. Occasionally, endometrial cancer can be diagnosed in asymptomatic women.

For ovarian cancer, the mean age at diagnosis is 63 years. Most women with epithelial ovarian cancer have symptoms prior to diagnosis. The most common symptoms include abdominal discomfort, abdominal swelling or bloating, urinary symptoms, and difficulty eating.

The most common symptoms of cervical cancer include post-coital or intermenstrual bleeding and vaginal discharge. Pelvic pain and urinary or bowel symptoms are uncommon in early stages of disease.

The majority of women diagnosed with vulval cancer present with a mass or an ulceration on the vulva. Vaginal bleeding and/or discharge are common symptoms in women with vaginal cancer. However, vaginal tumours can be asymptomatic and often are diagnosed during routine gynaecological examination.

Survival

For women diagnosed with endometrial, ovarian, and cervical cancer between 2003 and 2007 in England, the 5-year age-standardized relative survival is 75.9%, 40.8%, and 64.4%, respectively. The overall 5-year relative survival for women diagnosed with vulval and vaginal cancer in England and Wales between 1996 and 1999 was 58%.

Further reading

Bjorge T, Engeland A, Tretli S, Weiderpass E (2007). Body size in relation to cancer of the uterine corpus in 1 million Norwegian women. *International Journal of Cancer*, **120**, 378–83.

Cancer Research UK (2011). *CancerStats. Incidence 2008—UK*. Available at: <http://www.cancerresearchuk.org/prod_consump/groups/cr_common/@nre/@sta/documents/generalcontent/cr_072111.pdf>.

Schorge JO, Modesitt SC, Coleman RL, *et al.* (2010). SGO White Paper on ovarian cancer: etiology, screening and surveillance. *Gynecologic Oncology*, **119**, 7–17.

Walboomers JM, Jacobs MV, Manos MM, *et al.* (1999). Human papillomavirus is a necessary cause of invasive cervical cancer worldwide. *Journal of Pathology*, **189**, 12–19.

Key information for gynaecological cancers

	Age at presentation (years)	Screening	Treatment	Prognosis (5-year survival, %)
Uterine	70–74	No screening available	Surgery ± radiotherapy	75.9
Ovarian	80–84	No screening available	Surgery ± chemotherapy	40.8
Cervical	30–39	Cervical cytology	Surgery and/or chemoradiotherapy	64.4
Vulval/vaginal	>80	No screening available	Surgery ± radiotherapy	58.0

Management of vulval irritation and vulvodynia

Key learning points

Approximately 20% of women have experienced vulval symptoms

Cause is often multifactorial

Biopsy is not always indicated, unless a visible abnormality is present

Conservative management is usually successful

Consider involvement of dermatologist in difficult cases.

Definition

- Vulval irritation is a common condition that includes pruritus, pain, and changes in skin colour and texture
- Vulvodynia is vulval pain and/or discomfort occurring in the absence of gross anatomical or neurological findings. Symptoms include soreness, stinging, and/or a burning sensation
- Vulvodynia is classified into localized or generalized, according to the anatomical site of the pain, and whether the pain is provoked or unprovoked.

Epidemiology

- Community-based surveys indicate about one-fifth of women have significant vulval symptoms
- Different studies estimate prevalence of vulvodynia at around 15–18% of the adult female population
- Vulvodynia affects women of all ages but most commonly between 20 and 50 years.

Causes

Vulval irritation and/or pain can be caused by:

- Infections—herpes, Candida, etc.
- Vulval dermatoses—lichen sclerosus, lichen planus, contact dermatitis, psoriasis, plasma cell vulvitis, immunobullous disorders
- Hormonal deficiency—reduced levels of oestrogen in post-menopausal women
- Neurological—herpes neuralgia, pudendal nerve compression
- Pre-malignant conditions—vulval intraepithelial neoplasia (VIN)
- Malignancy—squamous cell carcinoma, Paget's disease
- Vulvodynia.

The cause of vulvodynia is usually multifactorial, but several theories have been proposed including:

- Embryologic abnormalities
- Genetic, immune, or hormonal factors
- Increased urinary oxalates or reduced pain threshold
- Infections, e.g. Candida or HPV
- Psychosexual causes, depression, or stress.

Clinical management

It is important to take a detailed history which should include:

- Adequate pain history to assess the degree of symptoms and the impact on the woman
- Medical, dermatological, and gynaecological history
- Any specific provoking factors and relation to intercourse
- Previous and current medications, and other forms of pain syndromes, e.g. fibromyalgia, interstitial cystitis, etc.
- Symptoms of urinary or faecal incontinence, as this can damage the vulval skin directly or indirectly by the use of sanitary products
- Personal or family history of autoimmune or atopic conditions
- The use of a questionnaire at the clinic can help to identify potential irritants.

Examination

- Careful and systematic examination, using adequate light
- Examine the vulva, vagina, cervix, and perianal region
- Examine the mouth and the skin of the rest of the body, e.g. elbows, scalp, nails, etc.

Investigations

- Common causes of vulval irritation can be diagnosed on clinical grounds
- Biopsies are required if there is clinical uncertainty, if the patient fails to respond to treatment, or if there is clinical suspicion of malignancy or VIN
- Biopsies are not necessary in the absence of a visible lesion
- Consider testing for thyroid disease, diabetes, and STDs, if clinically indicated
- Checking serum ferritin and skin patch testing should be performed if there are symptoms and/or signs suggestive of dermatitis
- Patients diagnosed with inflammatory conditions, e.g. lichen sclerosus or lichen planus, may benefit from testing for other autoimmune disorders if clinically indicated
- MRI is indicated for patients with symptoms suggestive of pudendal neuralgia.

Management

- Gentle care of the vulva is required
- Avoid potential irritants, e.g. perfumes, deodorants, wipes, detergents, shampoo, synthetic underwear, tight jeans, etc.
- Use soap substitutes, e.g. aqueous cream
- Low-oxalate diet may be helpful in some cases
- Adequate use of a suitable lubricant during intercourse
- If an STD is suspected, refer to GUM clinic for treatment and contact tracing
- Lichen sclerosus is usually treated with potent topical steroids, e.g. clobetasol propionate
- The gold standard for the treatment of VIN is local surgical excision. Reconstructive surgery may be needed after excision of large lesions
- Patients with urinary or faecal incontinence require adequate information regarding vulval hygiene and should be referred to the appropriate specialist clinics
- Patients diagnosed with vulvodynia should be given an adequate explanation of their diagnosis, relevant written information, and suggested contact information. Multidisciplinary approach is recommended. Clear instructions should be given on how to take medications and possible side effects. Contraindications and drug interaction with the patient's current medication should be assessed. Treatment may involve one or more of the following methods:
  - Topical therapy, e.g. lidocaine ointment, barrier petroleum jelly, steroids, topical nitroglycerin, topical amitriptyline, topical antifungals, capsaicin, etc. They should be used with caution to avoid the problem of irritancy
  - Low-oxalate diet, calcium citrate supplementation, and acupuncture may be helpful
  - Oral therapy, e.g. tricyclic antidepressants, SSRIs, anticonvulsants, etc.
  - Surgical management, e.g. local excision, vestibulectomy, perineoplasty, surgery for pudendal nerve entrapment, etc. Surgical treatment is suitable for a minority of patients and should be considered as the last resort
  - Biofeedback and physiotherapy. This is particularly helpful in patients with sex-related pain
  - Intravaginal electrical nerve stimulation (TENS)
  - Intralesion injections, using bupivacaine and steroids, have been successful for some patients. This can also be used for pudendal block
  - Interferon-alpha and botulinum toxin have been reported as successful treatments

- Psychosexual counselling and emotional support may be helpful, particularly with sex-related pain
- Involvement of a pain management team may be necessary in difficult cases.

Further reading

Dhar R and Nunns D (2009). Vulvodynia management. *Obstetrics, Gynaecology & Reproductive Medicine*, **19**, 175–7.

Neil S and Lewis F (2009). *Ridley's The vulva*, 3rd edn. Wiley-Blackwell, Chichester.

Royal College of Obstetricians and Gynaecologists (2011). *The management of vulval skin disorders*. Green-top guideline No. 58. Available at: <http://www.rcog.org.uk/womens-health/clinical-guidance/management-vulval-skin-disorders-green-top-58>.

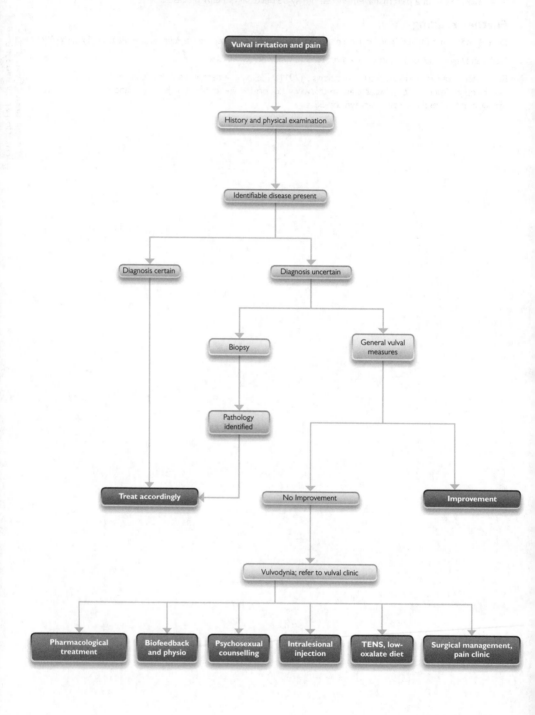

Algorithm for vulval irritation and vulvodynia

Vulval irritation and pain

History and physical examination

Identifiable disease present

Diagnosis certain

Diagnosis uncertain

Biopsy

General vulval measures

Pathology identified

Treat accordingly

No Improvement

Improvement

Vulvodynia; refer to vulval clinic

Pharmacological treatment

Biofeedback and physio

Psychosexual counselling

Intralesional injection

TENS, low-oxalate diet

Surgical management, pain clinic

Menopause and HRT

Definition

Menopause is defined as the LMP and is confirmed 12 months after the final menstruation. It is physiological, signifying the cessation of ovulation, falling serum oestradiol concentrations, and termination of reproductive capacity.

Common menopausal symptoms include vasomotor symptoms (hot flushes), sleeplessness, mood alteration, poor energy levels, impaired libido, and lower genital tract symptoms, including vaginal dryness.

Epidemiology

All women become menopausal, on average, between 50 and 51 years; however, symptom onset may be earlier and intermittent during the perimenopause. Seventy to 85% of menopausal women experience vasomotor symptoms; these are usually transient but may last for decades. Lower genital tract symptomatology has a slower onset.

Pathophysiology

The timing of menopause is predetermined genetically, and regular ovulation stops with the cessation of ovarian oestrogen production.

Oestrogen support is required for many purposes, including cerebral functions, bone homeostasis, cardiovascular function, and various effects on the skin and breast.

Vasomotor symptoms are thought to be caused by hypersensitivity to minor triggers, including temperature changes, alcohol, and caffeine.

Oestrogen exerts its effect on the vagina and lower urinary tract through improved cellular turnover and lubrication. Signs of poor vaginal oestrogenization include vaginal thinning, pallor, reduced elasticity, dryness, and easily traumatized epithelium.

Clinical management

Good clinical care of a woman who presents requesting help with managing her menopausal symptoms begins with thorough clinical assessment, including basic health checks and confirmation that she has engaged with all appropriate screening programmes. The clinician can then perform a basic risk assessment to inform the decisions about her treatment options. Important areas to assess include:

- Cardiovascular disease
- Osteoporosis
- Breast or other oestrogen-dependent neoplasia.

Vasomotor symptoms

After risk assessment, advice should be given concerning weight management, exercise, smoking, and intake of alcohol, caffeine, vitamin, and minerals. At this point, women may wish to see if these lifestyle measures help their symptoms.

If she then requests pharmacological intervention, the prescriber should be aware of the many possibilities for menopausal symptom treatment, but also to be certain of the patient's needs:

- Women with a family history of early-onset breast cancer would not be an appropriate candidate for oestrogen therapy as first-line treatment
- Women with existing low bone density may gain additional benefit from oestrogen
- Women with vaginal symptoms alone should receive local oestrogen.

Non-hormonal and non-prescribed pharmacological treatments

Most women expect to discuss non-hormonal treatments. The prescriber should be aware of complementary remedies (which may or may not be oestrogenic).

Available therapies with evidence include:

- Clonidine, a centrally active alpha-2 agonist, may help some women, but the evidence regarding its efficacy is of poor quality
- SSRI/SNRI drugs, including venlafaxine, fluoxetine, and desvenlafaxine, have a small, but significant effect, limited by short duration of efficacy and unwanted effects
- Gabapentin has been shown to reduce hot flushes in one study only and, therefore, requires further study
- Phytoestrogens (isoflavones and lignans) come from plants such as soy and red clover. The main isoflavones (genistein and daidzein) are present in beans, peas, red clover, and soybeans. The main lignans (enterolactone and enterodiol) are found in flaxseed, cereals, bran, and some fruits and vegetables. Due to the numerous preparations and relatively small study numbers, the evidence base is inconsistent and weak
- Black cohosh, an extract from a North American plant (*Actaea racemosa*) appears to relieve hot flushes through an unexplained mechanism. Again, data are conflicting, and there are concerns about safety, particularly with liver toxicity.

For the above preparations, the data do not generally stand rigorous scientific scrutiny with regard to their efficacy, and few studies have addressed safety. Red clover appears to have the strongest evidence base.

Hormonal therapies

HRT is indicated for the treatment of menopausal vasomotor symptoms when simple measures have failed and the patient is not considered at high risk of, or has had an, oestrogen-dependent neoplasia.

At present, in the UK, the Medical and Healthcare products Regulatory Agency (MHRA) continues to recommend that, if a woman wishes to take HRT, she should take the lowest effective dose for the shortest possible time, though the duration is not specified.

HRT may be prescribed as oestrogen-only treatment to women with a previous hysterectomy, or in women who retain their uterus as combined oestrogen-progestogen or tibolone. Many oestrogen preparations, combinations of oestrogen-progestogen preparations, and modes of delivery exist. Sequential combined HRT is usually biphasic, one half of a monthly cycle comprising oestrogen alone and the other oestrogen and progesterone, producing monthly bleeding. Continuous combined HRT contains the same daily mix of oestrogen and progesterone, without cyclical vaginal bleeding.

Systemic HRT is not indicated if the patient is experiencing symptoms of lower genital tract atrophy, as vaginal oestrogen preparations are effective, with few adverse effects.

Because HRT use has other beneficial effects on bone and potential risks to the breast and unclear long-term effects on the cardiovascular system, it is important to individualize therapy, according to the patient's needs and wishes.

An up-to-date knowledge of the management of menopause and its complications is vital for all prescribers. This aspect of women's health changes rapidly and attracts much attention from the lay and medical press.

Long-term treatment

If a woman wishes to continue long-term HRT, she should undergo regular health assessments, optimally every year, aiming to check that she is up to date for screening programmes, to confirm that the HRT she is taking has no new research data, and her therapy remains appropriate. The risk/benefit of her continuing treatment should be discussed and documented.

Further reading

Medical and Healthcare products Regulatory Agency (2007). *Hormone-replacement therapy: safety update.* UK public assessment report. Available at: <http://www.mhra.gov.uk/home/groups/pl-p/documents/websiteresources/con2032228.pdf>.

Royal College of Obstetricians and Gynaecologists (2010). *Alternatives to HRT for the management of symptoms of the menopause,* 2nd edn. Scientific impact paper No. 6. Available at: <http://www.rcog.org.uk/files/rcog-corp/uploaded-files/SIP_No_6.pdf>.

Santen RJ, Allred DC, Ardoin SP, *et al.* (2010). Postmenopausal hormone therapy: an Endocrine Society scientific statement. *Journal of Clinical Endocrinology & Metabolism,* **95** (Suppl 1), S1–66.

Suckling J, Lethaby A, Kennedy R (2006). Local oestrogen for vaginal atrophy in postmenopausal women. *Cochrane Database of Systematic Reviews,* **4**, CD001500.

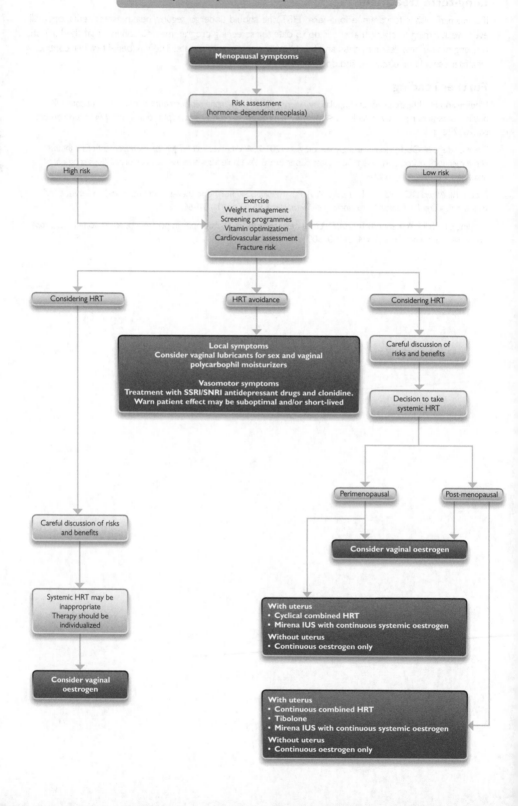

Care pathway for menopause and HRT

Menopausal symptoms

Risk assessment
(hormone-dependent neoplasia)

High risk

Low risk

Exercise
Weight management
Screening programmes
Vitamin optimization
Cardiovascular assessment
Fracture risk

Considering HRT

HRT avoidance

Considering HRT

Local symptoms
Consider vaginal lubricants for sex and vaginal
polycarbophil moisturizers

Vasomotor symptoms
Treatment with SSRI/SNRI antidepressant drugs and clonidine.
Warn patient effect may be suboptimal and/or short-lived

Careful discussion of
risks and benefits

Decision to take
systemic HRT

Perimenopausal

Post-menopausal

Careful discussion of risks
and benefits

Consider vaginal oestrogen

Systemic HRT may be
inappropriate
Therapy should be
individualized

With uterus
• Cyclical combined HRT
• Mirena IUS with continuous systemic oestrogen
Without uterus
• Continuous oestrogen only

**Consider vaginal
oestrogen**

With uterus
• Continuous combined HRT
• Tibolone
• Mirena IUS with continuous systemic oestrogen
Without uterus
• Continuous oestrogen only

SECTION 4

Gynaecology emergency presentations

Acute pelvic pain

Key learning points

Remember to take sexual and contraceptive history

Non-gynaecological causes of pelvic pain are common

Prompt evaluation is essential

Investigations should include pregnancy test, FBC, CRP, MSU, genital swabs, and imaging

TVS and further imaging, as needed.

Introduction

Acute pain generally has a well-defined onset, short duration, and defined aggravating and relieving factors and is usually associated with pathology.

History taking and examination are crucial in the diagnosis and management of women with pelvic pain. Localization of visceral pain is often difficult, as the uterus, cervix, and adnexae share the same visceral innervations as the lower ileum, sigmoid colon, and rectum. Because of this shared pathway, distinguishing between pain of gynaecological and GI origin is often difficult.

A critical component of management is to quickly identify the presence of conditions that are life-threatening such as severe haemorrhage from a ruptured ectopic pregnancy or impending perforation of an appendix.

History and examination should also consider infection of the urinary tract.

Common gynaecological causes

Mittelschmerz

This is pain in mid-cycle, occurring at the time of ovulation and more commonly seen in teenagers.

Dysmenorrhoea

Pain during menstruation that interferes with daily activities. Primary dysmenorrhoea is associated with release of prostaglandins during menstruation. This leads to uterine contraction, ischaemia, and pain. Secondary dysmenorrhoea is associated with presence of underlying pathology such as endometriosis, fibroids, or pelvic congestion.

Treatment

Antiprostaglandins, including naproxen or mefenamic acid, are effective in primary dysmenorrhoea. The COCP is highly effective, often in combination with NSAIDs.

Management of secondary dysmenorrhoea is usually through treatment of the underlying cause.

Acute pelvic inflammatory disease (PID)

PID occurs as a result of ascending infection from the endocervix, causing endometritis, salpingitis, tubo-ovarian abscess, and/or pelvic peritonitis. It is an important cause of acute pelvic pain, and its presence should be considered (see Chapter 80 on the management of acute pelvic infection).

Ovarian cysts

The ovary gives rise to a wide variety of tumours. During the reproductive years, the majority of ovarian masses are benign. The risk of malignancy is low. Benign tumours can be broadly divided into physiological and pathological cysts (see Chapters 77 and 78 on ovarian cysts).

Physiological cysts usually do not exceed 5 cm in size, are unilocular, and contain clear fluid.

Follicular cysts are the commonest and result from unruptured dominant follicles. They can achieve sizes of up to 10 cm. Small cysts are generally asymptomatic and resolve spontaneously.

A corpus luteum cyst is due to overactivity of the corpus luteum. It can be associated with pregnancy and usually disappears at around 12 weeks.

Complications of ovarian cysts

Large cysts can undergo torsion (twisting). As a result of this rotation, the blood supply to the ovary is occluded and can cause severe pain. Timely surgical intervention involves untwisting and removal of the cyst to prevent recurrence. Delayed action can result in ischaemic necrosis of the ovary.

Another complication is cyst rupture, causing intraperitoneal bleeding, chemical peritonitis, and pain. Rupture of endometriomata can also cause acute pain.

Management

In most cases, the treatment of an acute presentation of ovarian cysts depends on the cause of the pain (e.g. torsion or rupture) and nature of the cyst. If diagnosed as physiological, then it can be managed conservatively. Cases with resistant pain need surgery in the form of laparoscopy, proceeding to laparoscopic cystectomy or oophorectomy.

Management of abdominal pain in pregnancy is discussed in Chapter 30.

Further reading

Jurkovic D and Farquharson R (2011). *Acute gynaecology and early pregnancy*. RCOG Press, London.

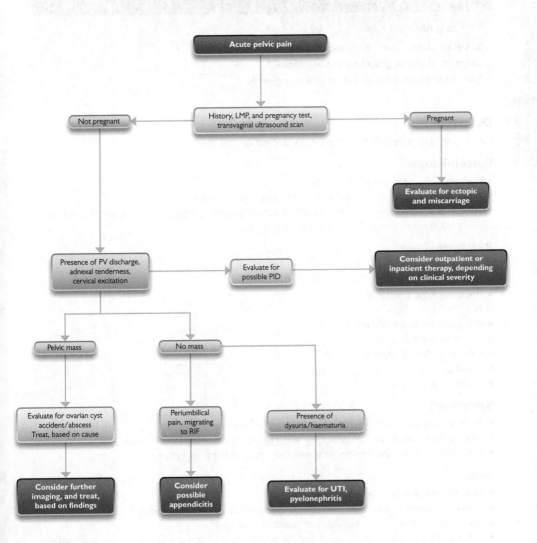

Algorithm for acute pelvic pain

Acute pelvic pain

History, LMP, and pregnancy test, transvaginal ultrasound scan

Not pregnant

Pregnant

Evaluate for ectopic and miscarriage

Presence of PV discharge, adnexal tenderness, cervical excitation

Evaluate for possible PID

Consider outpatient or inpatient therapy, depending on clinical severity

Pelvic mass

No mass

Evaluate for ovarian cyst accident/abscess Treat, based on cause

Periumbilical pain, migrating to RIF

Presence of dysuria/haematuria

Consider further imaging, and treat, based on findings

Consider possible appendicitis

Evaluate for UTI, pyelonephritis

Ectopic pregnancy

Key learning points

Be vigilant about ectopic pregnancy as a diagnosis

Diagnosis of ectopic pregnancy can be difficult

Role of expectant, medical, and surgical management.

Definition

Ectopic pregnancy is defined as a pregnancy located outside the uterine cavity.

Epidemiology

- Prevalence of ectopic pregnancy is 1.1%
- In the Early Pregnancy Assessment Unit (EPAU) population, the incidence is 3%
- The Fallopian tube is the most common site for ectopic pregnancy (95%). Other possible sites include interstitial, cervical, ovarian, C/S scar, and abdominal cavity.

Risk factors

- Previous PID
- Tubal surgery
- Previous ectopic pregnancy
- Infertility
- Assisted reproductive techniques
- Pregnancy with IUCD *in situ*
- Pregnancy after tubal ligation
- Smoking
- Maternal age >40 years.

Symptoms

- Amenorrhoea associated with vaginal bleeding and/or lower abdominal pain
- Vague GI symptoms in the form of nausea, vomiting, diarrhoea, or painful defecation
- Fainting/dizziness and shoulder pain, suggestive of ruptured ectopic pregnancy.

Signs

- Signs of peritonism on abdominal examination
- Adnexal tenderness and/or mass with cervical excitation during vaginal examination
- Signs of haemorrhagic shock, suggestive of ruptured ectopic
- However, the symptoms may be vague, and the patient may have no signs on examination. It is, therefore, essential to be highly suspicious of ectopic pregnancy.

Diagnosis

TVS is the imaging modality of choice for the diagnosis of ectopic pregnancy.

Ultrasound features

An empty uterine cavity with:

- Heterogenous adnexal mass
- Empty extrauterine sac with a hyperechoic ring ('doughnut' or 'bagel' sign)
- An extrauterine sac with a yolk sac or an embryo with or without a heart beat
- Free fluid in the pouch of Douglas
- Intrauterine pseudosac—collection of fluid or debris within the uterine cavity (in 5–20% of ectopics).

hCG assay

- An empty uterus when serum hCG is >1000 IU/L (discriminatory hCG level) is suggestive of an ectopic pregnancy
- Serial hCG levels, 48 h apart, may show plateauing of serum hCG or suboptimal rise or suboptimal fall.

Management

- Management depends on the clinical presentation, ultrasound findings, hCG level, and woman's preference
- Management options include expectant, medical, and surgical methods
- Expectant management is employed in a haemodynamically stable patient with a tubal mass <2 cm and serum hCG level <1000 IU/L, falling progressively
- Medical management is employed in a haemodynamically stable patient with a tubal mass <3.5 cm and serum hCG level <3000 IU/L
- In a stable patient, surgical management with a laparoscopic approach is preferable to an open approach
- The most expedient method should be employed in the presence of haemodynamic instability. This may be a laparotomy, and the method will depend on the surgeon's expertise
- Salpingectomy is the preferred surgical method in the presence of a healthy contralateral tube
- Salpingotomy should be considered in the presence of contralateral tubal disease and the desire for future fertility
- Appropriate counselling about the benefits and risks of each method is essential so that the woman can make an informed choice
- Non-sensitized women who are Rh-negative should receive anti-D immunoglobulin.

Further reading

American College of Obstetricians and Gynaecologists (2008). ACOG Practice Bulletin No. 94: Medical management of ectopic pregnancy. *Obstetrics and Gynecology*, **111**, 1479–85.

Association of Early Pregnancy Units (AEPU) (2007). *Guidelines 2007*. Available at: <http://earlypregnancy.org.uk/prof/documents/AEPUGuidelines2007.pdf>.

Confidential Enquiry into Maternal and Child Health (CEMACH) (2011). Saving Mothers' Lves: reviewing maternal deaths to make motherhood safer—2006–2008. The Eighth Report of the Confidential Enquiries into Maternal Deaths in the United Kingdom. *British Journal of Obstetrics and Gynaecology*, **118**, 1–203.

Royal College of Obstetricians and Gynaecologists (2004, reviewed 2010). *The management of tubal pregnancy*. Green-top guideline No. 21. Available at: <http://www.rcog.org.uk/files/rcog-corp/GTG21_230611.pdf>.

Algorithm for ectopic pregnancy

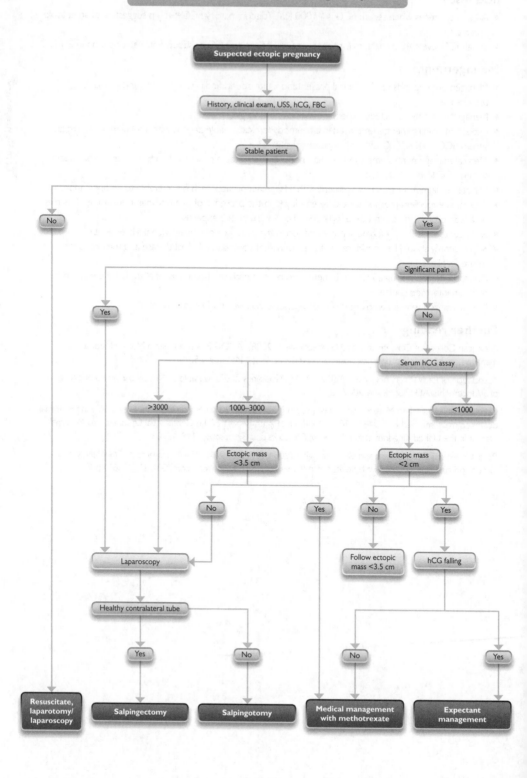

Miscarriage

Key learning points

One in five pregnancies miscarry

Consider pregnancy in a woman of reproductive age who presents with irregular bleeding

May present with severe bleeding, requiring prompt action

Do not forget administration of anti-D.

Definition

- Miscarriage is defined as the spontaneous loss of pregnancy before the fetus reaches viability, considered as 24 completed weeks of gestation
- Miscarriage can be classified as early (in the first trimester; up to 13 weeks' gestation) and late (in the second trimester; after 13 weeks up to 24 weeks' gestation).

Epidemiology

Once the pregnancy test is positive, there is around a 1:5 chance of having a miscarriage in the first 3 months. The risk of a second-trimester miscarriage is around 3%.

Causes of miscarriage

- Chromosomal abnormalities—the rate of chromosomal abnormalities increases with age
- Chronic maternal health factors—uncontrolled diabetes, severe hypertension, renal disease
- Infections (e.g. rubella, CMV, and mycoplasma, ureaplasma, Listeria, Toxoplasma infections)
- Trauma
- Anatomic factors—congenital or acquired anatomic factors such as cervical weakness.

Contributing factors

- Woman's age—the risk of early miscarriage increases with age. At the age of 30, the risk of miscarriage is 1 in 5 (20%). At the age of 42, the risk of miscarriage is 1 in 2 (50%)
- Lifestyle factors—smoking and heavy drinking are linked with miscarriage
- Chronic health problems, such as long-term medical conditions and chronic infection, may contribute to late miscarriage.

Presentation

- Women with spontaneous miscarriage usually present with cramping, abdominal pain, and vaginal bleeding
- The amount of bleeding can vary, from slight bleeding to severe and sometimes life-threatening
- Abdominal pain is usually located in the suprapubic area and may radiate to the lower back and thighs.

Presentation varies according to the category of miscarriage

- Threatened miscarriage—vaginal bleeding and/or abdominal/pelvic cramping during an ongoing pregnancy up to 24 weeks
- Complete miscarriage—woman may present with a history of bleeding, abdominal pain, and tissue passage. By the time the miscarriage is complete, bleeding and pain usually have subsided. Ultrasonography reveals an empty uterus
- Inevitable miscarriage—vaginal bleeding and pain. Products of conception emerge through the cervical canal, though nothing has been passed. Management is the same as incomplete miscarriage
- Incomplete miscarriage—vaginal bleeding may be intense and accompanied by abdominal pain. The cervical os may be open, with some products of conception already being passed. Ultrasonography is used to reveal whether some products of conception are still present in the uterus

- Missed miscarriage—when the woman may not be aware that the fetus has demised. May present with slight vaginal bleeding or may be detected at routine ultrasound examination.

Management

History

The patient's history should also include the following:

- Date of LMP
- Estimated length of gestation
- Bleeding disorders
- Previous miscarriage or termination of pregnancy
- Other symptoms, such as fever or chills, are more characteristic of an infection.

Note to consider any woman of childbearing age with vaginal bleeding pregnant until proven otherwise.

Examination

- Vital parameters—pulse, BP, pulse oximetry to assess haemodynamic stability
- Abdominal examination—size of uterus, tenderness, site of pain
- Pelvic examination—per speculum/vaginal examination to assess:
  - Bleeding from cervical os
  - Intensity of bleeding
  - Presence of clots or tissue fragments
  - Cervical motion tenderness (presence increases suspicion of ectopic pregnancy)
  - Status of internal cervical os—open indicates inevitable or possible incomplete miscarriage; closed indicates threatened miscarriage
  - Uterine size and tenderness, as well as adnexal tenderness or masses.

Investigations

- Blood group—Rh-negative women >12 weeks' gestation are administered anti-D to avoid Rh immunization
- FBC
- G & S or crossmatch
- TVS—to assess fetal viability if the cervical os is closed and to confirm complete miscarriage in the first trimester. Ultrasound diagnosis of missed miscarriage should only be considered with a mean gestational sac diameter ≥25 mm, with no obvious yolk sac, or with a fetal pole with crown rump length ≥7 mm, without evidence of fetal heart activity. Whenever in doubt, TVS is to be repeated after a week, prior to initiating medical or surgical treatment
- Abdominal ultrasound may be used in the second trimester
- β-hCG and serum progesterone are used, in conjunction with ultrasound, in cases of uncertain viability and to rule out an ectopic pregnancy. The level of β-hCG produced by a viable intrauterine pregnancy should normally increase by at least 66% every 48 h. The discriminatory level is the level of β-hCG at which one should see an intrauterine pregnancy on TVS. The level depends on expertise but, in most units, is considered as 1,500 IU/L. Using the combination of serial β-hCG and TVS, the diagnosis of ectopic pregnancy can be made with a sensitivity of 95–98% and a specificity of 98%
- A single measurement of serum progesterone is a helpful test. It will not help with the diagnosis of ectopic pregnancy, but it will help to differentiate between normal pregnancies and resolving ones (both intrauterine and ectopic).

Treatment

Complete miscarriage

- Check haemodynamically stable. May need fluid resuscitation/blood transfusion
- Start on iron supplement if anaemia detected
- Anti-D to be administered in Rh-negative women >12 weeks' gestation.

Incomplete miscarriage

Haemodynamically **unstable** patient/profuse per vaginal bleed:

- Fluid resuscitation/blood transfusion
- Urgent surgical evacuation
- Start on iron supplement if anaemia detected
- Anti-D to be administered in Rh-negative women.

Haemodynamically **stable** patient and without profuse bleeding and missed miscarriage:

Discuss options:

- Conservative management—await spontaneous expulsion of tissue or products of conception
  - Advantages—avoids anaesthesia, surgical complications
  - Disadvantage—may not be successful
- Medical management
  - With mifepristone and a prostaglandin-like misoprostol
  - Advantages—avoids anaesthesia, surgical complications
  - Disadvantage—may not be successful
- Surgical management.

Suction evacuation of the uterus is performed under general anaesthesia, and the indications are patients' preference for surgical method or failure of conservative or medical management of miscarriage.

In cases of incomplete miscarriage with heavy bleeding or suspicion of uterine sepsis, prompt evacuation of the uterus is necessary.

Risks include perforation of the uterus, infection, and incomplete evacuation.

Further reading

Abdallah Y, Daemen A, Kirk E, *et al.* (2011). Limitations of current definitions of miscarriage using mean gestational sac diameter and crown-rump length measurements: a multicenter observational study. *Ultrasound in Obstetrics and Gynecology*, **38**, 497–502.

RCOG Ultrasound Advisory Group (2011). *Addendum to GTG No 25 (Oct 2006): The management of early pregnancy loss.* Available at: <http://www.rcog.org.uk/files/rcog-corp/Addendum%20to%20GTG%20No%2025.pdf>.

Royal College of Obstetricians and Gynaecologists (2006). *The management of early pregnancy loss.* Green-top guideline No. 25. Available at: <http://www.rcog.org.uk/files/rcog-corp/uploaded-files/GT25ManagementofEarlyPregnancyLoss2006.pdf>.

Algorithm for miscarriage

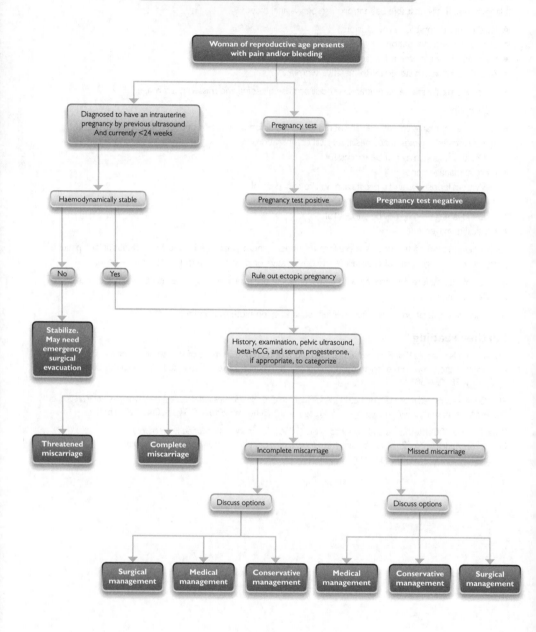

Management of ovarian masses in premenopausal women

Key learning points

Most ovarian masses in this age group are benign

Malignancy must be considered and appropriate tests performed prior to surgery

Conservative management is usually appropriate if criteria are met

Cysts >7 cm in diameter should undergo further imaging with MRI

Most cysts in pregnancy resolve spontaneously.

Introduction

During reproductive years, the majority of ovarian masses are benign, with the risk of malignancy being <1%. The incidence of ovarian cancer increases with advancing age. Ovarian cysts may be symptomatic, discovered incidentally, or detected through screening.

For history and examination, imaging with a pelvic mass, tumour markers, and risk of malignancy index, see Chapter 78 on the management of ovarian masses in post-menopausal women.

Additional tumour markers in premenopausal women

Ovarian germ cell tumours are more prevalent in women under 40 years; additional markers, if suspected, include:

- Alpha-fetoprotein (AFP): yolk sac tumour
- Lactate dehydrogenase (LDH): dysgerminoma
- Inhibin: granulosa cell tumour
- hCG: non-gestational ovarian choriocarcinoma.

Management

No further action required

- Simple ovarian cysts <5 cm
- These cysts are almost certainly benign.

Conservative management

- Ultrasound features are suggestive of a functional ovarian cyst
- Simple cysts ≤7 cm and normal CA-125
- Malignancy occurs in <1% (beyond 7 cm, papillary projections and intramural nodules may be overlooked, leading to the incorrect labelling of a cyst as 'simple'). Papillary projections within a unilocular cyst increase the risk of malignancy up to 6-fold and, therefore, should not be managed conservatively. Approximately 7% of 'simple' cysts >7 cm are borderline or malignant.

Or

- Risks of surgery outweigh the benefits of cyst removal
- Patient preference (after counselling regarding risks).

Follow-up of conservatively managed ovarian cysts

- Repeat USS at 3 months, with repeat CA-125 if cyst still present
- Over 50% of ovarian cysts detected in premenopausal women are functional, and 90% of functional cysts will have resolved within 2 months
- If the cyst has resolved, then no further follow-up is required
- If the cyst remains unchanged, an annual scan is recommended. There is no current evidence to determine the duration of follow–up, and some patients may prefer removal of the cyst

- Those cysts that increase in size or complexity should be considered for removal
- COCPs appear to be of no benefit for the treatment of functional ovarian cysts, although stopping progesterone methods may be useful.

Surgery

- Consideration of surgery should be made if the cyst does not meet the criteria for conservative management
- Risks, benefits, and potential complications of surgery should be individualized
- Conservative management may be appropriate in selected cases
- Indications for surgery:
  - Complex ovarian cysts (unless thought to be haemorrhagic or corpus luteum)
  - Simple cysts >7 cm. There is concern regarding accurate assessment of the cyst wall beyond 7 cm. If conservative management is preferred, an MRI of the cyst may be of value to characterize the cyst wall and exclude complex features
  - Symptomatic
  - Suspicion of malignancy.

Laparoscopic approach to surgical management

- Used when the risk of malignancy is considered to be low
- Thorough inspection of the peritoneal cavity should be performed
- If features suggestive of malignancy are encountered, a gynaecological oncologist should be consulted, regarding further evaluation and staging
- Ovarian cystectomy and preservation of ovarian tissue are preferred when surgery is performed for benign disease in women wishing to retain their fertility. The risk of oophorectomy, e.g. to control bleeding, should be mentioned during consent
- Women should be counselled preoperatively that, if features of malignancy are suspected during laparoscopy, then conversion to a full-staging laparotomy may be required.

Special situations

Endometrioma

- Can appear complex on ultrasound with a raised CA-125
- MRI can be useful
- Malignant transformation occurs in <1%, with the majority occurring in cysts >9 cm and in women >45 years
- Endometriomas should be managed within the spectrum of endometriosis and influenced by symptomatology. In general, conservatively managed endometriomas should be followed up with annual ultrasound. The development of solid elements should raise concern.

Pregnancy

- Incidence of 30% in first trimester, of which 90% represent corpus luteum of pregnancy and resolve spontaneously
- Majority can be managed conservatively
- Tumour markers tend to be elevated in pregnancy and are of limited use
- MRI may be useful when evaluating suspicious cysts
- Patients with suspicious adnexal masses detected during pregnancy should be discussed at the gynaecological oncology multidisciplinary team meeting
- Indications for conservative management:
  - Asymptomatic
  - Simple
  - <10 cm
  - If the cyst has not increased in size at the detailed 20-week scan, no further scan is necessary until 6 weeks post-partum

- Indications for surgery:
  - Complex cyst, with suspicion of malignancy
  - Increasing size
  - Symptoms suggestive of torsion, rupture, or bleeding
  - Surgery can be most safely performed early in the second trimester. In experienced hands, a laparoscopic approach appears safe
  - Ovarian cysts detected at C/S should be removed (cystectomy or oophorectomy), rather than aspirated, unless it is obviously functional when it should be left intact. Senior involvement is recommended.

Further reading

Leiserowitz GS, Xing G, Cress R, Brahmbhatt B, Dalrymple JL, Smith LH (2006). Adnexal masses in pregnancy: how often are they malignant? *Gynecologic Oncology*, **101**, 315–21.

Levine D, Brown DL, Andreotti RF, *et al.* (2010). Management of asymptomatic ovarian and other adnexal cysts imaged at US: Society of Radiologists in Ultrasound Consensus Conference Statement. *Radiology*, **256**, 943–54.

Royal College of Obstetricians and Gynaecologists (2011). *Management of suspected ovarian masses in premenopausal women*. Green-top guideline No. 62 (RCOG/BSGE joint guideline). Available at: <http://www.rcog.org.uk/files/rcog-corp/GTG62_021211_OvarianMasses.pdf>.

Algorithm for the management of ovarian masses in premenopausal women

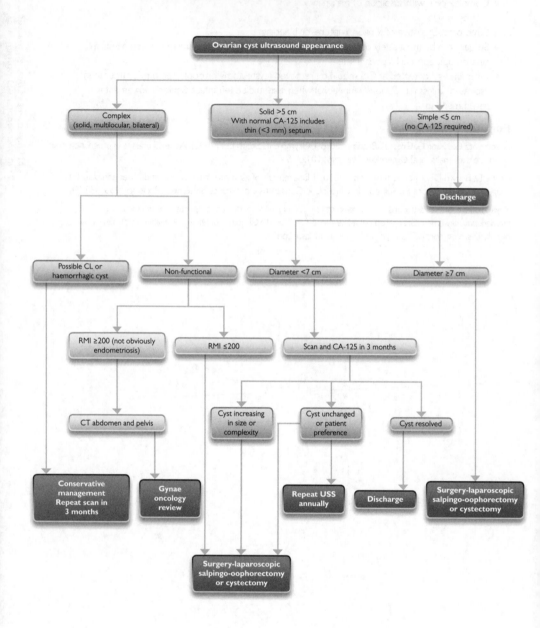

Management of ovarian masses in post-menopausal women

Key learning points

Ovarian cysts in a post-menopausal woman should be promptly investigated to exclude malignancy

Use of the 'risk of malignancy index' (RMI) can help to decide management pathway

Laparoscopic management is increasingly appropriate for cysts of borderline or low risk of malignancy.

Introduction

Approximately 20% of post-menopausal women will have abnormal ovarian morphology. Ovarian cysts may be symptomatic, discovered incidentally, or detected through screening.

History and examination

Symptoms have a very low predictive value for malignancy. In a recent study, seven symptoms were associated with ovarian cancer, including:

- Abdominal distension
- Urinary frequency
- Abdominal pain
- Post-menopausal bleeding
- Loss of appetite
- Rectal bleeding
- Abdominal bloating.

Family history relating to cancer predisposition syndromes should be sought, specifically ovarian, breast, endometrial, renal, and bowel cancer.

Clinical examination

- Unreliable
- Mobility, tenderness, and the presence of ascites are useful features to detect.

Imaging
Ultrasound examination

- The most valuable tool for initial evaluation
- TVS are more accurate than transabdominal
- Functional ovarian cysts are commonly unilateral, unilocular, and thin-walled. They usually measure <5 cm in diameter.

Sonographic characteristics associated with ovarian malignancy:

- Solid components, often nodular or papillary
- Septations, if present, that are thick (≥3 mm)
- Presence of ascites
- Peritoneal masses
- Enlarged lymph nodes.

Note unilocular cysts with a single thin (<3 mm) septum can be considered as simple.

MRI/CT/PET-CT

- If ultrasound cannot clearly characterize the nature of the adnexal mass, then further imaging studies should be considered
- No specific imaging modality has proved superior to others

- MRI allows accurate characterization of pelvic masses to determine the likely origin, i.e. uterine, ovarian, or bowel
- CT is more useful for staging a suspected ovarian cancer
- PET-CT yet to establish a clear role.

Tumour markers

CA-125

- Normal value <35 kU/L
- Elevated in 80% of women with ovarian cancer
- Elevated in only 50% of early-stage ovarian cancer
- Increased with conditions such as endometriosis, pelvic infection, fibroids, diverticulitis, inflammatory bowel disease, and hepatic dysfunction
- With elevated values, serial monitoring may be useful, since static high levels are less suspicious than rapidly rising levels.

HE4 (human epididymis protein 4)

- A novel marker yet to become widely used but may offer greater sensitivity and specificity when combined with CA-125.

Additional tumour markers

These may be useful if there is a possibility that the pelvic mass represents a metastasis from a separate primary cancer.

- Carcinoembryonic antigen (CEA): suspected colorectal primary
- CA 19-9: suspected colorectal and pancreatic primary
- CA 15-3: suspected breast primary.

Risk of malignancy index

- Clinical prediction tool, based on ultrasound, CA-125, and menopausal status to determine risk of malignancy from an adnexal mass
- Using RMI >200 gives a sensitivity of 78% and specificity of 87%
- Performs less well in premenopausal women due to the higher incidence of endometriomas, borderline, and non-epithelial tumours
- RMI > 200 needs to be discussed with a gynaecological oncologist.

$$RMI = U \times M \times CA\text{-}125$$

Where CA-125 = serum CA-125 in kU/L; M = menopausal status (M = 1 if premenopausal, and M = 3 if post-menopausal).

The ultrasound score (U) is calculated by awarding 1 point for each of the following characteristics:

- Multilocular cyst
- Evidence of solid areas
- Evidence of metastases
- Presence of ascites
- Bilateral lesions

U = 0, if none of the above listed features is found

U = 1, for ultrasound score of 1

U = 3, for ultrasound score ≥2.

Management

No further action required

- Post-menopausal simple ovarian cysts <1 cm
- These cysts are almost certainly benign.

Conservative management

- Ultrasound features are suggestive of a functional ovarian cyst (note functional ovarian cysts do not occur in late post-menopausal women)
- Post-menopausal simple cysts ≤5 cm and normal CA-125. The risk of malignancy is <1%.

Or

- Risks of surgery outweigh the benefits of cyst removal
- Patient preference (after counselling regarding risks).

Follow-up of conservatively managed ovarian cysts

Post-menopausal simple cysts:

- Ultrasound and CA-125 should be performed every 4 months for 1 year
- Those cysts that increase in size or complexity should be considered for removal.

Surgery

- Indications for surgery:
  - Complex ovarian cysts (unless thought to be haemorrhagic)
  - Post-menopausal simple cysts >5 cm. The risk of malignancy is thought to be 2–9%
  - Symptomatic
  - Suspicion of malignancy.

Laparoscopic approach to surgical management

- Used when the risk of malignancy is considered to be low
- Thorough inspection of the peritoneal cavity should be performed
- If features suggestive of malignancy are encountered, a gynaecological oncologist should be consulted
- Ovarian cysts in post-menopausal women should involve salpingo-oophorectomy (usually bilateral)
- Women should be counselled preoperatively that, if features of malignancy are suspected during laparoscopy, then conversion to a full-staging laparotomy may be required.

Aspiration of ovarian cysts

- Should not be performed routinely, since functional cysts will resolve spontaneously, neoplastic cysts will recur, and malignant cysts will be upstaged
- Image-guided aspiration can be considered if the cyst is causing significant symptoms and there are significant medical comorbidities contraindicating surgery
- If a cyst is aspirated, fluid should **not** be sent for cytology, as sensitivity and specificity are so poor as to render the result meaningless.

Further reading

Leiserowitz GS, Xing G, Cress R, Brahmbhatt B, Dalrymple JL, Smith LH (2006). Adnexal masses in pregnancy: how often are they malignant? *Gynecologic Oncology*, **101**, 315–21.

Levine D, Brown DL, Andreotti RF, et al. (2010). Management of asymptomatic ovarian and other adnexal cysts imaged at US: Society of Radiologists in Ultrasound Consensus Conference Statement. *Radiology*, **256**, 943–54.

Royal College of Obstetricians and Gynaecologists (2011). *Management of suspected ovarian masses in premenopausal women*. Green-top guideline No. 62 (RCOG/BSGE joint guideline). Available at: <http://www.rcog.org.uk/files/rcog-corp/GTG62_021211_OvarianMasses.pdf>.

Algorithm for the management of ovarian masses in post-menopausal women

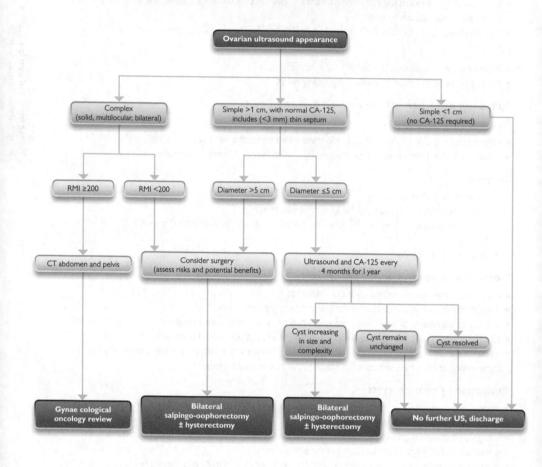

Management of vaginal discharge

Key learning points

Vaginal discharge is often physiological and may vary during the menstrual cycle

Infection must be excluded

If STI is diagnosed, referral to genitourinary services is required

Management is dependent on the cause.

Vaginal discharge can be defined as an alteration in genital secretions regarded as excessive or abnormal. Most women will experience a change in vaginal discharge at some time, and the likely cause will differ, according to her age, menstrual, and sexual history.

Aetiology

Physiological

The following are associated with alterations in physiological discharge:

- Menstrual cycle
- Ovulation
- Cervical ectropion
- Pregnancy
- Sexual arousal.

Vaginal infections

Vaginal infections are the most common cause of abnormal discharge.

Bacterial vaginosis

- At least 10% of woman of childbearing age have an overgrowth of predominantly anaerobic organisms in the vagina which results in bacterial vaginosis (BV)
- The discharge is characterized by an offensive smell and typically does not cause irritation or inflammation
- BV is associated with a decrease in the usually acidic environment of the vagina; douching, unprotected sexual intercourse, lubricants, excessive menses, and other factors increasing vaginal pH can be contributory in its development
- BV may resolve spontaneously and is not associated with complications if women are not pregnant or undergoing surgery
- The diagnosis can be made by microscopic examination of a Gram-stained slide of vaginal discharge or by taking a HVS
- Treatment is indicated if the woman is troubled by her symptoms, and options include a single oral dose of 2 g metronidazole or a 1-week course of intravaginal clindamycin 2% cream
- Recurrence of the condition is common, so women should be advised that the condition is generally harmless and how to modify any contributory factors.

Candidiasis

- 75% of women will experience candidal vulvovaginitis at least once in their lifetime. Up to 20% of women are asymptomatic vaginal carriers of Candida
- When symptomatic, common features are vulval itch, soreness, and vulvovaginitis
- The diagnosis can be made by microscopic examination of a Gram-stained slide of vaginal discharge or by taking a HVS
- For episodic infections, treatment with a single high-dose imidazole pessary (e.g. 500 mg clotrimazole) is recommended and is as efficacious as oral therapies
- Recurrent candidiasis is best treated with longer courses of imidazoles (e.g. miconazole 2% intravaginal cream daily, 78 g over 2 weeks), and underlying predisposing conditions should be considered

- Persistent vulval soreness after treatment is not uncommon, so advice on genital hygiene and the use of emollients, such as aqueous cream, can be given
- Candida is not a sexually transmitted infection, and, although symptoms may be exacerbated by sexual intercourse, treatment of sexual contacts does not affect relapse rates.

Trichomonas vaginalis (TV)

- This protozoal infection is sexually transmitted in adults and characterized by vulval soreness, frothy purulent discharge, vulvovaginitis, and a 'strawberry' cervix
- The diagnosis is made by microscopic examination of a wet preparation of vaginal discharge and by a Trichomonas-specific culture or molecular diagnostic test
- Although TV may be found on a HVS or cervical cytology sample, these tests have a low sensitivity for detecting TV
- Women in whom this infection is suspected should be referred to GUM
- Treatment with oral metronidazole is recommended; partner notification and treatment are essential.

Cervical infections

- Chlamydia
- Gonorrhoea
- Non-specific genital infection
- Herpes simplex virus.

Although the majority of chlamydial and gonorrhoeal infections do not cause symptoms in women, approximately one-third of those infected may notice an increase in vaginal discharge and/or post-coital bleeding because of cervicitis. Chlamydial infection is a common cause of discharge in sexually active woman under the age of 25 years. Non-specific genital infection similarly causes cervicitis and, along with Chlamydia and gonorrhoea, should be managed as a sexually transmissible infection. Herpes simplex infections can occasionally cause an intermittent cervicitis and discharge, even in the absence of vulval lesions.

Neoplasia

Neoplasia is not a common cause of vaginal discharge but should be considered if there is a bloodstained discharge and in the context of a woman's age, menstrual, and cytology history.

- Cervical polyps
- Genital wart
- Malignancy.

Miscellaneous

- Foreign body
- Streptococcal and staphylococcal vaginal infections
- Aerobic vaginitis
- Atrophic vaginitis
- Fistulae
- Rarely, pyometrium, dermatological causes, allergic causes, etc.

The possibility of multiple causes should always be considered.

Further reading

Public Health England (2002). *Management and laboratory diagnosis of abnormal vaginal discharge. Quick reference guide for primary care.* Available at: <http://www.hpa.org.uk/webc/HPAwebFile/HPAweb_C/1194947408846>.

Royal College of Obstetricians and Gynaecologists and British Association for Sexual Health and HIV (2006). The management of women of reproductive age attending non-genitourinary medicine settings complaining of vaginal discharge. *Journal of Family Planning and Reproductive Health Care,* **32,** 33–42.

Sherrard J, Donders G, White D (2011). 2011 *European (IUSTI/WHO) guideline on the management of vaginal discharge.* Available at: <http://www.iusti.org/regions/Europe/pdf/2011/Euro_Guidelines_Vaginal_Discharge_2011.Intl_Jrev.pdf>.

Care pathway for the management of vaginal discharge

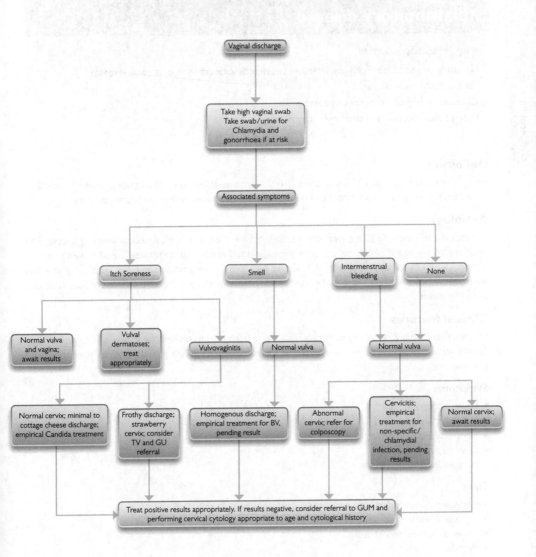

Management of acute pelvic infection/pelvic inflammatory disease

Key learning points

Normally due to acute ascending infection but may be exacerbation of chronic disease
Very variable presentation
Consider non-gynaecological diagnoses
Prompt identification and treatment important.

Definition

Pelvic inflammatory disease (PID) is an acute clinical syndrome associated with ascending spread of infection, usually from the vagina or cervix to the endometrium, fallopian tubes, and/or contiguous structures.

Aetiology

The majority of cases of PID are caused by sexually transmissible infections, especially in young people. The most commonly found pathogens are gonorrhoea and Chlamydia, although these are identified in only a quarter of PID cases diagnosed in the UK. Other bacteria, such as mycoplasmas, *Gardnerella vaginalis*, and anaerobes, which are often found in the vagina and some of which may be sexually transmissible, have also been implicated.

Clinical features

Women may have a wide variety of symptoms, ranging from mild to severe. Many cases of PID go unrecognized. Clinical criteria have been shown to give an accurate diagnosis in only 65–90% of cases when compared to laparoscopy.

Symptoms

- Lower abdominal pain
- Deep dyspareunia
- Abnormal vaginal bleeding
- Dysmenorrhoea
- Increased vaginal discharge.

Signs

- Cervical motion tenderness
- Adnexal tenderness
- Lower abdominal tenderness
- Pyrexia.

Investigations

- Chlamydia and gonorrhoea test
- Pregnancy test, if indicated
- MSU sample
- WBC, ESR, CRP
- Pelvic ultrasound and/or laparoscopy for severe cases and diagnostic uncertainty.

Complications

Short term

- Tubo-ovarian and pelvic abscesses
- Perihepatitis (Fitz-Hugh–Curtis syndrome).

Long term

- Ectopic pregnancy
- Infertility
- Chronic pelvic pain
- Deep dyspareunia.

Differential diagnosis

- Ectopic pregnancy
- Appendicitis
- UTI/pyelonephritis
- Endometriosis
- Complications of ovarian cyst
- Functional pain.

Management

As the sequelae of untreated PID may be serious, treatment should be instituted promptly in suspected cases. PID carries high morbidity; about 20% of affected women become infertile; 20% develop chronic pelvic pain, and 10% of those who conceive have an ectopic pregnancy.

Admission to hospital should be considered if symptoms are severe with systemic upset and when pelvic abscess and gynaecological/surgical emergencies are suspected. Rest and analgesia should be recommended, according to the severity of the disease.

Antibiotic treatment regimens should be effective against Chlamydia, anaerobes, and gonococci, if locally prevalent. IV therapy is indicated for severe disease.

Examples of treatment regimens

Oral ciprofloxacin 500 mg bd plus oral metronidazole 400 mg tds for 14 days.

Ceftriaxone 500 mg IM single dose, followed by oral doxycycline 100 mg bd and metronidazole 400 mg tds for 14 days.

Lack of response to therapy in severe infection or sustained peritonism may require imaging and/or laparoscopy to exclude and, where necessary, treat a potential pelvic abscess.

Women with PID, especially those under 25 years old and those with a new partner, should be advised not to have sex until sexual partners have been screened and treated as appropriate. It is estimated that the risk of the chronic complications of PID is doubled by a further episode of infection; hence, the avoidance of re-infection is of paramount importance. Partner management and the future use of barrier contraception will significantly reduce the risk of further PID.

Follow-up should be arranged to review adherence and response to treatment, abstinence, partner management, and the possible development of complications.

Further reading

British Association of Sexual Health and HIV Clinical Effectiveness Group (2011). *UK national guideline for the management of pelvic inflammatory disease 2011*. Available at: <http://www.bashh.org/documents/3572.pdf>.

Algorithm for the management of acute pelvic infection and PID

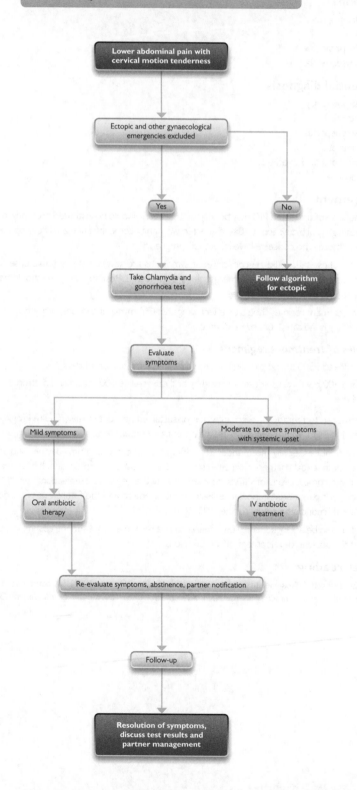

Ovarian hyperstimulation syndrome (OHSS)

Key learning points

A potentially serious complication of ovarian superovulation

OHSS does not occur in the absence of hCG

Most complications occur as a result of significant fluid shifts

Management is usually supportive but may include delay or cancellation of cycle.

Definition

OHSS is a serious iatrogenic complication of ovarian superovulation. It is a systemic disease, caused by the presence of vasoactive products released by the hyperstimulated ovaries.

Incidence

- One in three IVF cycles have mild forms of OHSS
- 6% of cycles are complicated by moderate or severe OHSS
- Occurs after any form of supraphysiological ovarian stimulation, including after using clomifene citrate, but is more common after the use of injectable gonadotrophins for ovulation induction.

Pathophysiology

- OHSS represents an exaggerated response to ovarian stimulation
- The exact aetiological factor remains unknown
- The syndrome is dependent on the presence of hCG, since OHSS does not occur if hCG is withheld
- Ongoing hCG stimulation by early pregnancy is a significant risk factor for the development of severe OHSS
- Numerous vasoactive substances produced by the ovaries have been implicated in the pathophysiology of the disease, including PGs, inhibin, vascular endothelial growth factor (VEGF), tumor necrosis factor alpha, and insulin-like growth factor 1, leading to increased capillary permeability and leakage of protein-rich fluid from the vascular compartment, third-space fluid accumulation, haemoconcentration, and intravascular volume depletion
- Life-threatening complications with OHSS include vascular thrombosis, renal and liver dysfunction, and ARDS.

Risk factors

- Age <30 years
- Low BMI
- PCOS and/or high AMH level
- The use of the GnRH long downregulation protocol for ovarian stimulation
- High serum oestradiol (>9000 pmol/L) on the day of hCG injection
- Rapidly rising oestradiol levels (>50% from previous day)
- hCG administration for oocyte maturation or in the luteal phase
- Large number of oocytes retrieved (20 or more)
- Pregnancy and, especially, multiple pregnancy.

Diagnosis

The typical symptoms of OHSS include:

- Abdominal distension, sense of abdominal bloatedness, and pain
- Nausea and vomiting
- Oliguria in advanced cases
- Differential diagnoses include a complicated ovarian cyst (ovarian torsion, or cyst haemorrhage or rupture), ectopic pregnancy, pelvic infection, intra-abdominal haemorrhage, and appendicitis.

For the purpose of prognosis, OHSS can be divided into 'early' and 'late'.

- **Early OHSS** usually presents within 9 days of the hCG injection and reflects excessive ovarian response to the exogenous hCG injection administered for final follicular maturation
- **Late OHSS** presents 9 days after the hCG injection and almost always reflects endogenous hCG stimulation from an early pregnancy. Late OHSS tends to be more severe and longer-lasting than early OHSS.

The severity of OHSS can be divided into three grades:

- **Mild:**
  1. Mild abdominal pain and bloating
  2. Ovarian size is usually <8 cm in average diameter
  3. Minimal ascites on TV scanning
  4. Blood tests are usually normal
- **Moderate:**
  1. Increased abdominal distension
  2. May be associated with nausea and vomiting
  3. Ovarian size >8 cm in diameter
  4. Ascites can be detected on abdominal scanning in most cases
- **Severe:**
  1. Increasing abdominal distension and pain
  2. Oliguria is common
  3. Ascites, with or without right-sided hydrothorax, can be clinically detected and is often tense
  4. Evidence of haemoconcentration (haematocrit >45%), low albumin level, abnormal liver and renal functions, and hyponatraemia secondary to increased antidiuretic hormone release.

Management of OHSS

- OHSS is a self-limiting condition
- Spontaneously resolves within 2 weeks in most cases
- Aim to provide symptomatic relief and avoid complications.

Prevention is preferred to treatment of OHSS.

Identify risk factors, and apply the following strategies to minimize the risk.

Cycle cancellation before hCG injection

- Cancel treatment cycle by discontinuation of gonadotrophin
- Withhold hCG injection
- Review of the stimulation protocol before starting a new IVF cycle.

Coasting

- Coasting involves withholding of gonadotrophin injections for ovarian stimulation for 1 or more days to allow FSH, and consequently oestradiol, levels to fall to a safe level (<2500 pg/mL or 9000 pmol/L) before administering hCG
- Coasting could reduce the number of oocytes retrieved if the oestradiol level drops to a low level.

Elective cryopreservation of all embryos

- Avoid pregnancy by embryo replacement at a later date
- This strategy aims to prevent a late-onset OHSS but will not reduce the risk of early OHSS.

Cabergoline

- It binds to VEGF receptors in the vascular epithelium and reduces capillary permeability and the risk of OHSS
- Dose: 2–4 mg, given over a course of 7–8 days, starting on the day of either hCG injection or oocyte retrieval.

GnRH agonist trigger

The use of the GnRH agonist in an antagonist ovarian stimulation cycle, in order to reduce the risk of OHSS, has been investigated. The GnRH agonist has a shorter half-life, compared to the hCG injection, and may, therefore, result in a lower risk of OHSS. However, its use could also be associated with a lower clinical pregnancy rate after IVF.

For details of management, see Algorithm.

1. NSAIDs should be avoided, as they could further compromise renal function in patients with OHSS
2. Diuretics should be avoided, as they could aggravate hypovolaemia
3. A slow rate of ascitic fluid drainage should be followed, in order to avoid cardiovascular collapse from massive fluid shifts. In most cases, a maximum of 1.5 L of ascitic fluid could be drained per 24 h.

Further reading

Huang JYJ and Rosenwaks Z (2010). Preventive strategies of ovarian hyperstimulation syndrome. *Journal of Experimental & Clinical Medicine*, **2**, 53–62.

National Collaborating Centre for Women's and Children's Health; commissioned by the National Institute for Clinical Excellence (2004). *Fertility: assessment and treatment for people with fertility problems*. Clinical guideline, February 2004. Available at: <http://www.nice.org.uk/nicemedia/pdf/cg011fullguideline.pdf>.

Royal College of Obstetricians and Gynaecologists (2006). *The management of ovarian hyperstimulation syndrome*. Green-top guideline No. 5. Available at: <http://www.rcog.org.uk/files/rcog-corp/GTG5_230611.pdf>.

Algorithm for ovarian hyperstimulation syndrome

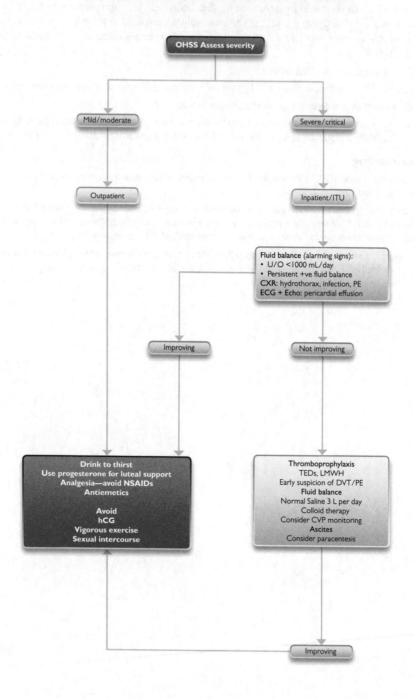

OHSS Assess severity

Mild/moderate

Severe/critical

Outpatient

Inpatient/ITU

Fluid balance (alarming signs):
- U/O <1000 mL/day
- Persistent +ve fluid balance
CXR: hydrothorax, infection, PE
ECG + Echo: pericardial effusion

Improving

Not improving

Drink to thirst
Use progesterone for luteal support
Analgesia—avoid NSAIDs
Antiemetics

Avoid
hCG
Vigorous exercise
Sexual intercourse

Thromboprophylaxis
TEDs, LMWH
Early suspicion of DVT/PE
Fluid balance
Normal Saline 3 L per day
Colloid therapy
Consider CVP monitoring
Ascites
Consider paracentesis

Improving

Emergency contraception

Key learning points

Emergency contraception (EC) is an effective means of pregnancy prevention after unprotected intercourse

Both hormonal and non-hormonal means are effective

Following administration of EC, pregnancy tests should be performed after 3 weeks if a period has not started

Screening for STIs should be offered.

Introduction

There is clear evidence that giving emergency post-coital contraception reduces the chance of pregnancy from a recent episode of UPSI or failed contraception. However, epidemiological studies have failed to show that improving access to EC has any effect on pregnancy or termination of pregnancy rates. It is, therefore, important in these consultations to discuss/encourage/provide ongoing regular and more reliable contraception as well as providing EC. The risk of STIs should be considered, and screening for STI should be included in these consultations.

Non-hormonal EC

The most effective form of EC is the insertion of a copper intrauterine device (Cu IUD). If retained, it provides very effective ongoing contraception. It should be offered as an option to all women, but, if it cannot be fitted straightaway, hormonal EC should be given. All those providing EC should know where to refer for IUD fitting if they are not able to do the fitting themselves. The device can be fitted up to 120 h after the first episode of UPSI within that cycle or up to 5 days after predicted ovulation in women who have reasonably regular menstrual cycles.

Hormonal EC

There are two forms of hormonal EC.

- LNG 1.5 mg is licensed for use up to 72 h after UPSI, and there is some evidence to show its efficacy up to 96 h
- Ulipristal acetate 30 mg (UPA) has become available, and this is licensed to 120 h after UPSI.

There is clear evidence that UPA is more effective than LNG after 72 h. LNG is often recommended up to 72 h as it is less expensive, but patients should be given the choice.

LNG is a very safe medication, with no absolute contraindications; the dose should be doubled to 3 mg if the patient is also taking (or has taken in the last 4 weeks) enzyme-inducing medication such as carbamazepine, ritonavir, or St John's wort.

UPA is not recommended if the woman is taking enzyme-inducing medication, antacid medication, proton pump inhibitors, or H2 receptor antagonists. It should not be used if she has severe asthma not controlled by glucocorticoids or if there is a risk that she might already be pregnant from UPSI >120 h ago but within the current menstrual cycle.

After EC

Pregnancy tests can take up to 3 weeks to become positive after an episode of UPSI. If there have been several episodes of UPSI earlier in that menstrual cycle, it may be helpful to do a pregnancy test, but, if it is negative, the patient should be advised that they might already be pregnant. It would be acceptable to give LNG in these circumstances to reduce the risk of pregnancy from later UPSI episodes in the cycle.

Rarely, vomiting may occur shortly after hormonal EC is given. In these circumstances, a further dose can be given after an antiemetic. A pregnancy test 3 weeks later should be advised if a normal period has not occurred or if there is any other concern that she might be pregnant.

Further reading

Faculty of Sexual and Reproductive Health Clinical Effectiveness Unit (2011). *Emergency contraception*. Available at: <http://www.fsrh.org/pages/clinical_guidance.asp>.

Raymond E, Trussell J, Polis C (2007). Population effect of increased access to emergency contraceptive pills: a systematic Review. *Obstetrics and Gynecology*, **109**, 181–8.

Algorithm for emergency contraception

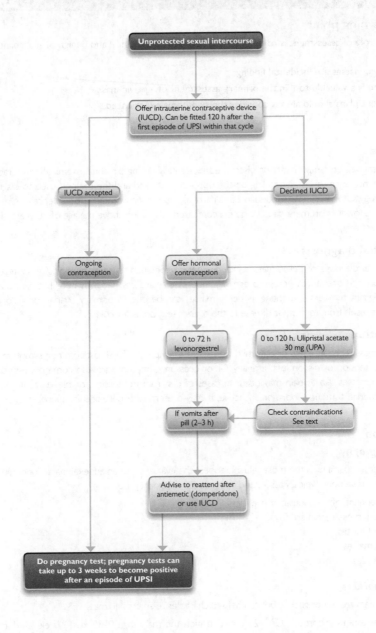

Pelvic mass

Key learning points

The main role of assessment is to differentiate between physiological and benign or malignant pathology

Many pelvic masses are incidental findings

Ultrasound is a valuable tool in the primary assessment of a pelvic mass

Management plans should always consider the symptoms experienced.

Incidence

A pelvic mass may be symptomatic or discovered incidentally during bimanual examination or radiological imaging. The incidence varies, depending on the population studied and the method used to diagnose the pelvic pathology. Ovarian cysts are found in 2.5–31% of asymptomatic women. The incidence of symptomatic ovarian cysts is lower in premenopausal women, compared to women above the age of 50 years (1:1000 vs 3:1000, respectively).

Differential diagnosis

The differential diagnosis of pelvic masses includes benign conditions such as physiological cysts, endometrioma, mature cystic teratoma, ectopic pregnancy, tubo-ovarian abscess, pedunculated fibroid, or diverticular disease. Malignant tumours presenting as pelvic masses can be due to primary ovarian or Fallopian tube carcinoma or result from metastatic disease to the ovaries (e.g. breast or colon).

Presentation

Most pelvic masses produce few or only mild, non-specific symptoms. The most common symptoms include abdominal distension or discomfort. Urinary, GI, or pressure symptoms are also common, especially with large ovarian masses. Acute pain may occur in cases of cyst rupture, torsion, or bleeding into an ovarian cyst. If the ovarian tumour is hormonally active, it may present with oestrogenic, androgenic, or virilizing symptoms.

Evaluation

Ultrasonography

Greyscale ultrasonography is the most valuable tool in the evaluation of an adnexal mass. Sonographic characteristics that have been typically associated with ovarian malignancy are:

- Solid component, often nodular or papillary
- Septations, if present, that are thick (>2–3 mm)
- Presence of ascites
- Peritoneal masses
- Enlarged nodes.

Tumour markers

Tumour markers are not diagnostic but can help to characterize an ovarian mass.

CA-125: the serum glycoprotein CA-125 concentration (normal range 0–35 kU/L) is elevated in 80% of women with ovarian cancer. However, the levels can be within the normal range in 50% of women with stage I disease. Serum CA-125 is also increased in patients with benign gynaecological conditions (endometriosis, PID, leiomyomata), non-gynaecological conditions (diverticular disease, ascites, pleural effusion), and other malignancies such as epithelial ovarian, colon, or breast cancer.

Serum levels of AFP, hCG, and LDH should be measured in all women under the age of 40 years found to have a complex ovarian cyst on ultrasonography, due to higher prevalence of germ cell tumours in younger women.

Management

Factors that should be considered when making decisions regarding the management of ovarian masses include: presence of symptoms, risk of malignancy, age of the patient, future fertility issues, and presence of comorbidities that may impact on patient's fitness for surgery.

It is recommended that an 'RMI' should be used to select those women who require primary surgery in a cancer centre by a gynaecological oncologist.

The RMI is a clinical prediction rule, based on ultrasound, CA-125, and menopausal status data, discussed in Chapters 77 and 78.

Premenopausal women

Simple ovarian cysts measuring <5 cm do not require any treatment or follow-up. The use of COCPs appears to be of no benefit, and these cysts are likely to resolve within three menstrual cycles. Women with simple cysts measuring between 5 and 7 cm should have yearly ultrasound follow-up. For women with simple cysts measuring >7 cm, either additional imaging (MRI) or surgical treatment should be considered, because these cannot be assessed completely by ultrasonography.

For women with complex ovarian masses or ultrasound features suggestive of malignancy, surgery is recommended. Depending on the patient's preferences and fertility aims, the surgery may involve unilateral or bilateral salpingo-oophorectomy, collection of fluid for peritoneal cytology, inspection and biopsy from the peritoneal surfaces, omental biopsy, appendicectomy, and para-aortic lymph node sampling. Surgery can be performed via a laparoscopic or an open approach.

Surgery is also indicated in cases where ovarian cyst torsion is suspected, in order to relieve the symptoms and prevent infectious complications. The removal of the affected ovary is the treatment of choice in these cases.

Post-menopausal women

Simple, unilateral, unilocular ovarian cysts, <5 cm in diameter, have a low risk of malignancy and, in the presence of a normal serum CA-125 levels, can be managed conservatively. USS and measurement of serum levels of CA-125 should be performed every 4 months. If there is no change in the size of the cyst or the cyst has resolved after 1 year of follow-up, then the patient can be discharged from follow-up.

Women at intermediate risk of malignancy (RMI <200) can be suitable for laparoscopic surgery. Laparoscopic management of ovarian cysts in post-menopausal women should involve oophorectomy (usually bilateral), rather than cystectomy.

Women at high risk of malignancy (usually RMI >200 or clinical suspicion) need to be managed by a gynaecological oncologist in a cancer centre. The aim of surgery in these cases is to confirm the diagnosis, to assess the extent of the disease, and to attempt optimal debulking. The laparotomy should be performed through a midline incision and include: collection of peritoneal fluid for cytology, bilateral salpingo-oophorectomy and hysterectomy, omentectomy, appendicectomy, biopsies from any suspicious peritoneal surfaces, and para-aortic lymph node sampling.

Pregnant women

The majority of women with an ovarian mass during pregnancy can be managed conservatively. If surgery is necessary, then it can be performed early in the second trimester. Surgery in pregnancy does not appear to increase the rate of congenital abnormalities or unexplained stillbirths. An ovarian cyst diagnosed at the time of a C/S should be removed, rather than aspirated, as malignancy may be missed.

Further reading

Levine D, Brown DL, Andreotti RF, et al. (2010). Management of asymptomatic ovarian and other adnexal cysts imaged at US: Society of Radiologists in Ultrasound Consensus Conference Statement. Radiology, 256, 943–4.

Mazze RI and Kallen B (1989). Reproductive outcome after anesthesia and operation during pregnancy: a registry study of 5405 cases. *American Journal of Obstetrics & Gynecology*, **161**, 1178–85.

Royal College of Obstetricians and Gynaecologists (2003). *Ovarian cysts in postmenopausal women*. Green-top guideline No. 34. Available at: <http://www.rcog.org.uk/files/rcog-corp/GTG34OvarianCysts.pdf>.

Royal College of Obstetricians and Gynaecologists (2011). *Management of suspected ovarian masses in premenopausal women*. Green-top guideline No. 62. Available at: <http://www.rcog.org.uk/files/rcog-corp/GTG62_021211_OvarianMasses.pdf>.

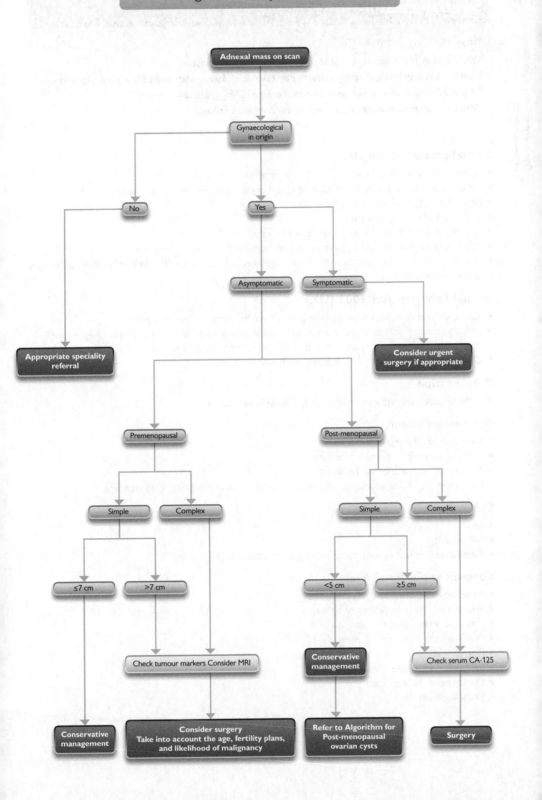

Algorithm for pelvic mass

Adnexal mass on scan

Gynaecological in origin

No → Appropriate speciality referral

Yes

Asymptomatic

Symptomatic → Consider urgent surgery if appropriate

Premenopausal

Post-menopausal

Simple

Complex

Simple

Complex

≤7 cm

>7 cm

<5 cm

≥5 cm

Check tumour markers Consider MRI

Conservative management

Check serum CA-125

Conservative management

Consider surgery
Take into account the age, fertility plans, and likelihood of malignancy

Refer to Algorithm for Post-menopausal ovarian cysts

Surgery

Sexual assault

Key learning points

Sexual assault is defined as acts of sexual touching without consent

Presentation may be significantly delayed, may take many forms, and present in differing locations

Early involvement of a sexual assault referral centre (SARC) is vital

Contact children's services in cases where children are involved.

Sexual assault in the UK

- The lifetime risk of sexual assault is 1 in 4–6 for women
- It is estimated that only one in five adult rapes is reported (i.e. prevalence much higher)
- One in ten victims of sexual assault are men
- 12% of assaults are by strangers
- 45% are by acquaintances and 43% by intimate partners
- 45% involve vaginal rape, 10% anal rape, 15% oral rape, and 25% digital penetration
- The incidence of child sexual abuse is unknown. Possibly, only one in 20–50 assaults of children are known to supervising authorities.

Sexual Offences Act 2003 (UK)

- Rape is defined as non-consensual penetration of mouth, vagina, or anus by a penis
- Sexual assaults are acts of sexual touching without consent. Sexual assault by penetration involves the insertion of object or body parts, other than the penis, into the vagina or anus
- Children under 13 cannot legally consent to any sexual activity.

Presentation

This can be acute/delayed/acute on chronic (particularly for children).

Acute sexual assault

- Sixteen to 58% have genital injuries
- Thirty-eight to 80% have non-genital injuries
- May present to A & E or via the police
- May present to GUM/gynaecological/psychiatric services, with covert or overt symptoms.

Delayed

- GUM
- Gynaecology
- Antenatally (increase in domestic violence and assault during pregnancy).

Concerns arising for children

- Repeated A & E attendances
- Poor parent-child interactions or behaviour
- Child known to social services
- Any injuries to child under 1 year
- Domestic abuse
- Explanation inconsistent with injuries
- Disclosure of abuse by child
- Delay in presentation.

Initial assessment

- When the event occurred
- What sexual act or acts occurred
- Whether she gave, and/or whether she was competent to give, consent
- Whether she has reported, or wants to report, to the police
- What her immediate medical needs are.

Ring the local SARC for advice, or discuss with the on-call consultant for emergency medicine or gynaecologist and/or trained sexual assault police officer if no SARC.

Consider use of an early evidence kit (should be available in all emergency departments) for samples from mouth (wash and swab) and urine.

Assess competence so an appropriate adult and/or interpreter can be arranged for in a timely manner.

History

- Details of alleged assault, description of assailant, meeting place, place of assault
- Times since assault; when ate, drank, showered/bathed/douched, passed urine, opened bowels, changed clothes
- Ingestion of any kind of drugs or alcohol
- Gynaecological, obstetric, and sexual history
- LMP, menstrual cycle, contraception
- Basic medical, surgical, and psychiatric history
- Use of prescribed medications; over-the-counter, social, recreational drugs
- Social history, including family circumstances, children, support.

Examination: key points to record

- Demeanour/intoxication/psychological state
- Height/weight (calculate BMI)/handedness (right/left)
- General observations: BP, pulse, skin conditions, scars
- Injuries using body diagrams: description of injury, dimensions, exact location in relation to bony landmarks
  - Describe as petechiae, abrasion, laceration, incision, bruise. Do NOT give opinion as to causation (although can suggest consistent with typical injuries, e.g. fingertips or typical defence injuries)
- Genital/anal examination: describe any injury and relevant negatives
- Describe hymen (hymenal remnants), as appropriate
- Oral examination: describe any injury to mucosa, teeth, tongue.

Remember to consider keeping clothes and any object, such as tampon, condom, or diaphragm, as these may be useful as evidence that may harbour DNA. Locard's principle—every contact leaves a trace—determines evidence collection.

Forensic samples to be taken/considered after sexual assault

- Skin, fingernails, hands, perioral neck, lower abdomen, and other relevant sites (i.e. contact sites—determined by history of assault)
- All skin swabs are double, i.e. one wet and one dry, as this has been shown to yield the most DNA
- Mouth swab and mouthwash
- Buccal swabs are taken for victim DNA
- Vagina vulval/perineal swabs (× 2)
- Low vaginal swabs (× 2)
- With Cusco's speculum: HVS (× 2) and endocervical swabs (× 2)
- Swab from speculum (× 1)
- Anus/perianal swabs (× 2)

- With proctoscope: anal swabs (x 2)
- Rectal swabs (x 2).

Time frames for finding DNA samples

- Mouth samples <48 h
- Skin samples <48 h
- Samples after digital penetration <12 h
- Anal samples <72 h
- Vaginal samples <7 days
- Blood for toxicology <72 h
- Urine for toxicology <14 days
- Documentation of injuries <21 days.

Recent assaults within 14 days should ideally be discussed with a SARC, even if the person does not want police involvement. There are a variety of arrangements for disclosure of details that are possible so the police can be involved at a later date or data shared between police forces on an anonymous basis, if wished.

'Historical' assault, including of children, can be assessed in any setting, but gathering of evidence is different to acute reporting. With children, the presence of some STIs may imply sexual abuse. These include gonorrhoea over the age of 1 year, Chlamydia over 3, and syphilis and HIV at any age if congenital infection excluded.

In acute cases, maintaining the chain of evidence is crucial, or it may be that any evidence obtained may not be used in a subsequent court case.

Further reading

Dalton M (2004). *Forensic gynaecology: towards better care for the female victim of sexual assault.* RCOG Press, London.

Care pathways for sexual assault

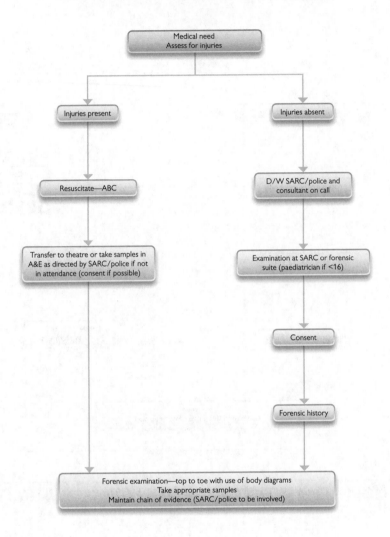

Medical need
Assess for injuries

Injuries present

Injuries absent

Resuscitate—ABC

D/W SARC/police and consultant on call

Transfer to theatre or take samples in A&E as directed by SARC/police if not in attendance (consent if possible)

Examination at SARC or forensic suite (paediatrician if <16)

Consent

Forensic history

Forensic examination—top to toe with use of body diagrams
Take appropriate samples
Maintain chain of evidence (SARC/police to be involved)

Care pathways for sexual assault

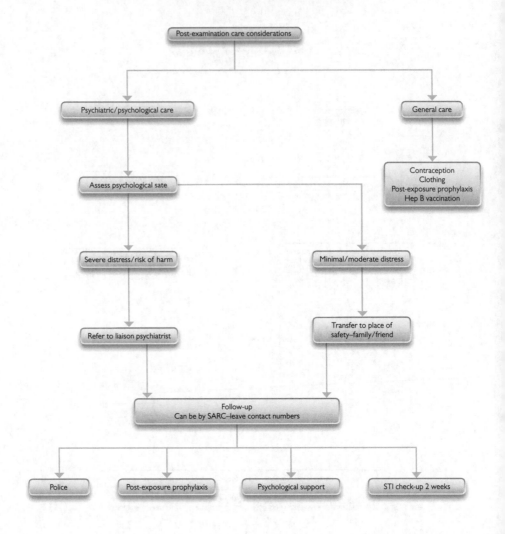

INDEX